KT-528-550

OXFORD MEDICAL PUBLICATIONS

Ophthalmic Anaesthesia

www.bma.org.uk/library

Oxford Specialist Handbooks published and forthcoming

Oxford Specialist Handbooks in Anaesthesia
Ophthalmic Anaesthesia

Edited by

Professor Chandra M. Kumar

Department of Anaesthesia
Khoo Teck Puat Hospital
Yishun, Singapore

Professor Chris Dodds

Department of Anaesthesia
The James Cook University Hospital
Middlesbrough, UK

Professor Steven Gayer

Professor of Anaesthesiology and Ophthalmology
Bascom Palmer Eye Institute
University of Miami Miller School of Medicine
Miami, USA

OXFORD
UNIVERSITY PRESS

OXFORD
UNIVERSITY PRESS

Great Clarendon Street, Oxford OX2 6DP

Oxford University Press is a department of the University of Oxford.
It furthers the University's objective of excellence in research, scholarship,
and education by publishing worldwide in

Oxford New York

Auckland Cape Town Dar es Salaam Hong Kong Karachi
Kuala Lumpur Madrid Melbourne Mexico City Nairobi
New Delhi Shanghai Taipei Toronto

With offices in

Argentina Austria Brazil Chile Czech Republic France Greece
Guatemala Hungary Italy Japan Poland Portugal Singapore
South Korea Switzerland Thailand Turkey Ukraine Vietnam

Oxford is a registered trade mark of Oxford University Press
in the UK and in certain other countries

Published in the United States
by Oxford University Press Inc., New York

British Library Cataloguing in Publication Data
Data available

Library of Congress Cataloging-in-Publication-Data
Data available

Typeset by Cenveo, Bangalore, India
Printed in Great Britain
on acid-free paper by
Ashford Colour Press Ltd, Gosport, Hampshire

ISBN 978-0-19-959139-8

10 9 8 7 6 5 4 3 2 1

Preface

A comprehensive knowledge of ophthalmic anaesthesia is essential for anaesthetists, ophthalmologists and all those who are involved in the care of patients undergoing eye and orbital surgery. This book is intended to provide both basic and detailed understanding of anatomy, physiology, pharmacology, specific anaesthetic techniques, and the principles related to the safe conduct of general and regional anaesthesia in children and adults undergoing ophthalmic surgery. The changes that have occurred in the field over the last decades are also emphasized.

The contributors of this book are internationally known, respected clinicians and academicians from the United Kingdom, France, India, Singapore, the United States and elsewhere, who have had a pronounced influence in the evolution of ophthalmic anaesthesia. Collectively, they have presented lectures and conducted workshops throughout the populated continents. They have edited journals and texts, performed laboratory and clinical research, authored peer-reviewed articles, book chapters, and more. They have advanced the field, disseminated their knowledge, and made ophthalmic anaesthesia a safer specialty.

This book is dedicated to ophthalmic anaesthetists, ophthalmologists, nurses and those who care for ophthalmic patients worldwide.

Editors
Chandra M. Kumar
Chris Dodds
Steven Gayer

Contents

Contributors

Dr K. G. AuEong
Senior Consultant Ophthalmologist
Singapore International Eye
Cataract Retina Centre,
Singapore

Dr Joanna Budd
Consultant Anaesthetist
Worcestershire Royal Infirmary
Worcester, UK

Dr Benjamin Chang
Consultant Ophthalmologist
Department of Ophthalmology
and Visual Sciences
Khoo Teck Puat Hospital,
Singapore

Mr Imtiaz A. Chaudhry
Senior Academic Consultant,
Oculoplastic and Orbit Division
King Khaled Eye Specialist Hospital
Riyadh, Saudi Arabia

Dr Anjolie Chhabra
Associate Professor of Anaesthesia
All India Institute of Medical
Sciences
New Delhi, India

Professor Chris Dodds
Department of Anaesthesia
The James Cook University
Hospital
Middlesbrough, UK

Mr Tom Eke
Consultant Ophthalmologist,
Department of
Ophthalmology, Norfolk &
Norwich University Hospital
Norwich, UK

Dr Marc Allan Feldman
Head, Section of Anesthesia
Cole Eye Institute
Departments of General
Anesthesia and Outcomes
Research
Cleveland Clinic
Cleveland, USA

Dr Irina Gasanova
Assistant Professor of
Anesthesiology and Pain
Management
Director of Postanesthesia Care
Unit and Day Surgery
University of Texas
Southwestern Medical Center
Dallas, USA

Professor Steven Gayer
Professor of Anaesthesiology and
Ophthalmology
Bascom Palmer Eye Institute
University of Miami Miller School
of Medicine
Miami, USA

Dr R. W. Johnson
Retired Consultant Anaesthetist
Bristol, UK

Professor Girish P. Joshi
Professor of Anesthesiology and
Pain Management
Director of Perioperative Medicine
and Ambulatory Anesthesia
University of Texas
Texas, USA

Dr Chin Wui Kin
Department of Ophthalmology
and Visual Sciences
Khoo Teck Puat Hospital,
Singapore

Dr K.-L. Kong
Consultant Anaesthetist
Department of Anaesthesia
City Hospital
Birmingham, UK

Professor Chandra M. Kumar
Department of Anaesthesia
Khoo Teck Puat Hospital
Yishun, Singapore

Dr Kathryn McGoldrick
Professor and Chair
New York Medical College
Department of Anaesthesiology
Valhalla
New York, USA ·

Dr Hamish McLure
Consultant Anaesthetist
Department of Anaesthesia
St James' University Hospital
Leeds, UK

Dr Howard Palte
Assistant Professor of
Anaesthesiology
University of Miami Miller School
of Medicine
Miami, USA

Professor Jacques Ripart
Division Anesthésie Réanimation
Douleur Urgence
GHU Caremeau
Nimes, France

Dr Tiakumzuk Sangtam
Department of Ophthalmology
and Visual Sciences
Khoo Teck Puat Hospital
Singapore

Dr Ashish Sinha
Assistant Professor of
Anesthesiology & Critical Care
Assistant University of
Pennsylvania School of Medicine
Philadelphia, USA

Dr Jacquiline Tuttiven
Assistant Professor of
Anaesthesiology
University of Miami Miller School
of Medicine
Miami, USA

Dr Edwin Xavier Vicioso
New York Medical College
Department of Anaesthesiology
Valhalla
New York, USA

Dr Shashi Vohra
Consultant Anaesthetist
Department of Anaesthesia
City Hospital
Birmingham, UK

Abbreviations

❶	proceed with caution
ACC/AHA	American College of Cardiology/American Heart Association
ADHD	attention deficit hyperactivity disorder
ASA	American Society of Anesthesiologists
BBB	blood–brain barrier
BIS	bispectral index
BMI	body mass index
BP	blood pressure
BPH	benign prostatic hypertrophy
bpm	beats per minute
C_3F_8	octafluoropropane
CHF	congestive heart failure
CN	cranial nerve
CNS	central nervous system
COPD	chronic obstructive pulmonary disease
COX-2	cyclo-oxygenase
CSF	cerebrospinal fluid
CT	computed tomography
CVA	cerebrovascular accident
CVP	central venous pressure
DCR	dacryocystorhinostomy
DSEK	Descemet's stripping endothelial keratoplasty
DVT	deep vein thrombosis
ECCE	extra-capsular cataract extraction
ECG	electrocardiogram
EEG	electroencephalogram
EMG	electromyograph
EMLA	eutatic mixture of local anaesthetic
EOM	extra-ocular muscle
ERG	electroretinography
$ETCO_2$	end tidal carbon dioxide
ETT	endotracheal intubation
EUA	evaluations under anaesthesia
FDT	forced duction test
GA	general anaesthetic
GABA	gamma-aminobutyric acid

GI	gastrointestinal
GOR	gastrooesophageal reflux
GTN	glycerine tri nitrate
h	hours
H_2	histamine receptor
HCL	hydrogen chloride
HIV	human immunodeficiency virus
ICD	implantable cardiac defibrillator
IM	intramuscular
iNOS	inducible nitric oxide synthetase
INR	international normalized ratio
IOP	intra-ocular pressure
IPPV	intermittent positive pressure ventilation
IV	intravenous
LA	local anaesthetic
LASIK	laser *in-situ* keratomileusis
LMA	laryngeal mask airway
m	minutes
MAC	minimum alveolar concentration
MAC	monitored anaesthesia care
MAOI	monoamine oxidase inhibitor
MH	malignant hyperpyrexia
MI	myocardial infarction
MMR	masseter muscle rigidity
MRI	magnetic resonance imaging
mV	millivolt
Na/KATPase	sodium-potassium adenosine triphosphatase
NICU	neonatal intensive care unit
NK_1	neurokinin 1
NMB	neuromuscular blocker
NPO	nil by mouth
NSAIDs	non-steroidal anti-inflammatory drugs
OA	orbital axis
OCR	oculo-cardiac reflex
OSA	obstructive sleep apnoea
PABA	para-amino benzoic acid
$PaCO_2$	pulmonary arterial carbon dioxide tension
PACU	post-anaesthesia care unit
PALS	paediatric advanced life support (a training programme)
PCA	patient-controlled analgesia

PDNV	post-discharge nausea and vomiting
PONV	postoperative nausea and vomiting
PPV	positive pressure ventilation
PR	per rectal
RA	regional anaesthesia
RCT	randomized controlled trial
REM	rapid eye movement
ROP	retinopathy of prematurity
RP	retinitis pigmentosa
RSI	rapid sequence induction
RVO	retinal vascular occlusion
SC	subcutaneously
SCH	suprachoroidal haemorrhage
SF_6	sulfur hexafluoride
SVTs	supraventricular tachycardias
TCI	target-controlled infusion
TIVA	total intravenous anaesthesia
TMJ	temporomandibular joint disorder
TT	tracheal tube
VA	visual acuity
VA	visual axis
VAS	visual analogue scale
VR	vitreoretinal
WHO	World Health Organization

Chapter 1

History of ophthalmic anaesthesia

Dr Robert W. Johnson

Introduction

Advances in anaesthesia may result from a number of factors. Serendipity, curiosity or inspiration may sometimes be responsible but drug discovery, increased knowledge of physiology and anatomy, technological advances and changing expectations of patients, surgeons, and society in general have perhaps been most important in the evolution of ophthalmic anaesthesia. Of course, all such advances require individuals with insight, energy, and perseverance to recognize potential and develop the advance.

As stated by Louis Pasteur in 1854, 'In the field of observation, chance only favours the prepared mind.' Sometimes changes in anaesthesia have of necessity followed surgical technical advances and at others, advances in anaesthesia have facilitated surgical developments.

The most tolerant of surgeons inevitably seek anaesthesia that permits their procedures to be undertaken under ideal conditions and with minimal morbidity and mortality. Similarly, less invasive and faster surgical techniques, such as modern small-incision phacoemulsification cataract surgery, have encouraged anaesthetic technique development suited to high throughput and ambulatory surgery.

It is traditional to concentrate on individuals and their contributions but in this chapter it is intended to dwell as much on the stimulus for development as the undoubted qualities of those who recognized potential and undertook the necessary investigative and developmental processes. It is not always safe to assume that the first recorded observation of an advance was made by the person to whom history attaches attribution.

Topical anaesthesia

Topical anaesthesia

Cocaine has a long history and its transition from social, religious, and mystical use to medical purposes is documented from 1653. Almost complete cessation of use of cocaine in medicine (apart from nasal surgery in some countries) resulted from its significant adverse effects including toxicity and addiction and the development of safer and more effective topical and injectable drugs.

Following isolation and purification reported by Niemann in 1855, Koller's demonstration in 1884 of the anaesthetic effect of topical cocaine to abolish the pain for ophthalmic surgery was a major advance. At this time the disadvantages of ether-based general anaesthesia were considerable and a valid alternative was welcomed by surgeons and patients alike.

Cocaine, in its initial concentration and technique of use, was shown to cause hazing and damage to the cornea. Some questioned its use for ophthalmic surgery.

By 1901 Koller repeatedly instilled cocaine into the eyes of rabbits keeping one eye closed and the other open. Opacity only occurred in the open eye, encouraging care when using topical anaesthesia to ensure continuous maintenance of corneal hydration with tears or other suitable replacement. Allen suggested using dilute cocaine to precede strong cocaine to prevent most of the burning and stinging associated with its instillation: this was especially important in the traumatized eye.

Topical application of cocaine was only effective for brief, superficial surgery. Topical cocaine did not diffuse deep enough to totally abolish sensation from the iris in most patients and did not abolish pain resulting from extra-ocular muscle traction or the cutting of the optic nerve, even when placed next to the globe through incisions in the bulbar conjunctiva by Turnbull.

In 1884, Knapp achieved anaesthesia during more invasive operations using multiple subconjunctival injections of cocaine around the muscles and optic nerve.

- Despite sedatives and morphine, many patients continued to have pain and would squeeze their eyelids, impeding surgery and raising intra-ocular pressure. The problem was overcome with the addition of orbicularis muscle akinesia by a facial nerve block that was introduced by van Lint and later modified by Wright and O'Brien (see 📖 Facial nerve block, p. 102).
- However, as a result of pain, many patients would still strain and move about, compromising the surgical field. Heavy sedation was used to control this activity, often started the day before surgery and continued through the prolonged convalescence. Such anaesthesia was used for the majority of patients having cataract surgery through the 1930s.
- Topical cocaine was gradually replaced by tetracaine (amethocaine) 1% in the 1930s, even though the new drug did not dilate the pupil or provide the vasoconstriction of cocaine. Later replacements included proparacaine in the 1960s and then ibuprocaine, lidocaine, and bupivacaine in the 1990s. Unlike cocaine, the safety of the newer topical anaesthetics has been tested according to contemporary standards.

- Topical anaesthesia for cataract surgery gradually declined after the late 1930s and did not reappear significantly for cataract surgery until the last two decades, encouraged by the advent of minimally invasive surgery (see Timeline, p. 124).

Injection anaesthesia techniques

Injection of cocaine into the orbit was the logical extension of a purely topical approach enabling pain reduction from the deeper structures and provision of akinesia of the globe. Knapp reported such injections soon after the report of Koller's discovery of the topical effectiveness of cocaine and after observing that topical, subconjunctival, and subcutaneous injections were inadequate to block deeper pain (1884). Cocaine caused relatively little pain on injection, produced excellent vasoconstriction, and blocked sensory and motor nerves.

However, local anaesthetic (LA) injection in the orbit was slow to gain acceptance because large-volume orbital injection often caused pain and side effects such as syncope, cold sweats, and hallucinations, which were rare with topical administration of cocaine. In addition, some patients still experienced pain during surgery. In the first published reports of cocaine injection for enucleation in the United States, Knapp reported syncope with 0.37cc of 2% cocaine. He described forced traction on the globe following which the patient experienced vasovagal syncope. Knapp interpreted this reaction, probably incorrectly, as 'toxicity of cocaine in the vascular orbit'.

As a result, use of minimal volumes of cocaine in the orbit became established. Failure to recognize or differentiate systemic or local toxicity from the vasomotor effects of painful injection, oculocardiac reflex (see 📖 Oculo-cardiac reflex, p. 44) from muscle traction and pain from non-anaesthetized areas, established a false picture of orbital regional anaesthesia.

Morbidity and poor operating and postoperative recovery conditions using general anaesthesia (GA) with ether caused Elschnig and Lowenstein to persist in developing LA techniques for enucleation and other deep eye surgery. They were able to achieve success using nerve block with cocaine and epinephrine injected in the area of the ciliary ganglion with spread of anaesthetic to the optic nerve sheath, the nearby oculomotor and nasociliary nerves, and to the sensory nerves of the conjunctiva, proving that a total block could be done with less than half the accepted toxic dose of cocaine. A similar technique was used for cataract surgery. Direct block of the facial nerve was a useful adjunct to prevent inadvertent eye closure and to decrease pressure of the muscles on the globe.

Thus by the 1920s it was established that good surgical conditions for cataract surgery as well as for enucleation could be safely provided by regional orbital block, which was then called 'ciliary ganglion block', although many other nerves were blocked in addition. Gifford, in the USA, recognized that those who had adopted ciliary ganglion block had a high frequency of excellent surgical results (1935).

The major proponent of ciliary ganglion block, facial block, and globe paresis for cataract surgery in the US was Atkinson, who reported his technique and its benefits on a number of occasions.

- Atkinson's intraconal ciliary ganglion block became known as the 'retrobulbar block' (see 📖 Traditional appellations, p. 84). The success of the intraconal block led to the explosion of regional anaesthesia for cataract surgery in the 1940s and 50s. At this time the majority of these blocks were performed by the surgeon in the US, with GA remaining the predominant method in many other parts of the world. Some patients still had pain and would strain at the wrong time from inadequate single-needle injection of 'retrobulbar' anaesthesia, and some patients would not develop akinesia, which led some US surgeons to return to general anaesthesia.

Local anaesthetic agents and adjuvants

- **Epinephrine**: when added to cocaine, was found to extend useful anaesthesia time with cocaine, decrease vitreous pressure, decrease bleeding, and decrease the dose needed. Because cocaine worked even better when epinephrine was added, the search for an 'ideal' ophthalmic LA gained little momentum.
- **Procaine** (originally named novocaine): cocaine was replaced by procaine after 1905 in general surgery because it was safer. Procaine became more effective when epinephrine was added to obtain vasoconstriction resulting in more satisfactory anaesthesia, but only gradually replaced cocaine in ophthalmology because of cocaine's familiarity. Procaine eventually became the standard LA agent for injection in ophthalmology. Procaine was non-addictive, more stable in solution, had a longer shelf life, and could be purchased in bottles ready for use. Cocaine had to be prepared almost daily by the pharmacist to be reliable, and drug laws required strict record keeping.

  The concept of injection of minimal volumes of LA for eye surgery, based upon the early clinical observations of cocaine and procaine/ epinephrine mixtures, delayed the more rational use of procaine and the other LA drugs that followed.

  The concentration of epinephrine in the final procaine/epinephrine solution ranged from 1:1,000 to 1:5,000. Many patients, perhaps not surprisingly, exhibited toxic reactions to this combination when injected in the orbit in any but the smallest quantity. Larger quantities could cause syncope and cold sweats similar to that reported with cocaine.

- **Hyaluronidase:** techniques using small amounts of procaine (and large amounts of sedation) would have remained the techniques of choice for cataract surgery, but for Atkinson's report in 1949 that larger doses of LA to produce akinesia could be injected within the cone if hyaluronidase was injected along with it and if the globe was massaged to disperse excess fluid. His recommended dose of 2% procaine in the muscle cone for cataract surgery went up from 1cc in 1934 to 1–1.5cc in 1949 after the addition of hyaluronidase, and even higher subsequently. Procaine use persisted until the introduction of the less toxic lidocaine in 1940, which required less epinephrine and could also be mixed with hyaluronidase. Atkinson encouraged the use of lidocaine and the recommended volume of local increased to the amount producing noticeable proptosis, 2–3cc in 1955 and 4cc or more up to 8cc in 1964. The combination of hyaluronidase, larger anaesthetic volume, and prolonged, deliberate pressure over the orbit (oculocompression) was shown by Kirsch to produce the hypotony of the globe desired for ideal intracapsular cataract extraction. Over the years, development of newer LA drugs encouraged the search for single agents or drug combinations, with or without epinephrine, that would provide the desired safety and anaesthetic conditions (speed of onset, duration and quality of anaesthesia, motor block) for surgery of various types and durations (see 📖 Hyaluronidase p. 64).

There remains much variation in the favoured LA drug menu and no doubt this will evolve yet further.

- 1905: novocaine (later named procaine)
- 1943: lidocaine
- 1957: mepivacaine and bupivacaine (marketed 1965)
- 1969: prilocaine
- 1972: etidocaine and articaine
- 1996: ropivacaine

Other considerations

Improved drugs were an important advance but complications also occurred from accidental penetration or perforation of the globe and development of safer orbital block procedures followed (see 📖 Modified intraconal block, p. 89). In addition, the move to outpatient surgery discouraged use of long-acting sedatives. Thus painless block technique and an orbital block that removed the need for a separate, often painful, facial nerve block for orbicularis control were desirable goals.

The danger of injection deep into the orbital apex had been known for 100 years as a cause of blindness and even death, irrespective of the insertion point of the needle or needle design. Most surgeons tried to prevent these disasters by applying knowledge of orbital anatomy, but Atkinson and Gifford additionally extolled the use of specially prepared dull needles. Even though the optic nerve and central artery could not be perforated with such dull needles in dogs in the laboratory, human cases still occurred. As a result, the use of anaesthesia personnel in the ophthalmic surgery theatre became logical to sedate, monitor, and resuscitate patients as needed.

It was also sensible and appropriate that anaesthetists should undertake orbital blocks provided they were trained in ophthalmic LA. The guidelines for LA for cataract surgery published in 1993 jointly by the Royal College of Anaesthetists and the College of Ophthalmologists (UK), while far from perfect, raised awareness of the risks of LA and their avoidance.

Brainstem anaesthesia could occur with any LA drug but was more frequent with large-volume injections and longer needles placed quite deeply within the orbit (see 📖 Central nervous system spread and brainstem anaesthesia, p. 348). The potential pathway was demonstrated for anaesthetic to enter the midbrain via the orbital extension of the meninges covering of the optic nerve sheath. Dynamic CT scans by Unsold showed that the optic nerve and central retinal artery moved about in the orbit and could be placed in the pathway of needles during movement of the eye when asking the patient to 'look up and in' as then recommended by Atkinson. Furthermore, the globe could be seen rotating its posterior pole in the direction opposite to the anterior hemisphere when digital pressure was applied to elevate the anterior globe in an attempt to provide more 'safe space' for inferior needle insertion. Thus it was discovered that the optic nerve was placed at more risk of injury than was previously believed.

Katsev measured the orbits of many humans and showed that orbital lengths vary considerably; demonstrating that the commonly used 1½in needle could reach dangerous areas of the orbital apex in 15–20% of patients, regardless of the approach of the orbital block. Techniques were described in the 1980s to eliminate penetration of the optic nerve sheath and needle damage to the optic nerve and the central retinal artery. These were based on the pre-1970s concept of the anatomy of the orbit that considered the orbit to be divided into two compartments: an intraconal space contained by the extra-ocular muscles and intermuscular septum and an extraconal space or the space between the bony orbit and the intraconal space (see 📖 Intraconal versus extraconal blocks, p. 86).

Injections to provide anaesthesia for orbital surgery were then described as being safer when placed in the extraconal space by Davis, Bloomberg (1986) and Weiss (1989) and just as effective as intraconal injections. These safer spaces were named peribulbar by Davis or peri-ocular by Bloomberg or Weiss. It was correct that injections made into this space could produce anaesthesia and akinesia, but how could LA placed outside the muscle cone penetrate inside the muscle cone to block the intraconal nerves to the globe and extra-ocular muscles?

A Dutch anatomist and ophthalmologist, Koornneef, made anatomical reconstructions of the human orbit from a large number of specimens of many ages which showed that there was no complete 'intermuscular septum' dividing the orbit into intraconal and extraconal compartments, except near the insertion of the muscles to the globe, or deep in the orbital apex. There were adipose tissue compartments between the muscles through which anaesthetic drugs could move in the orbit and could readily anaesthetize intraconal nerves.

Newer techniques using this information were described in the late 1980s and 1990s by Hustead, Hamilton, Fanning and others allowing needles to be placed more safely into the muscle cone with the eye in primary or upward gaze without reaching the optic nerve or orbital apex provided that appropriate sites of insertion, correct trajectories, and appropriate needle lengths were used (see 📖 Needle considerations, p. 92). These techniques did place needles further away from the optic nerve and required larger volumes to be injected for effectiveness than either Atkinson's intraconal or Gifford's apical techniques. They also took longer to produce anaesthesia and akinesia.

The volume of injectate recommended for the new techniques varied from 3–10cc using either a single injection or multiple injections into 'safe areas'. The safe areas described included more anteriorly in the cone than the standard injection of Atkinson, and with the eyes straight ahead as described by Gills and Loyd or Hamilton, or above the eye as by Kelman and Thornton, into the lateral cone as in the block by Gills and Loyd, outside the cone in the anterior peribulbar sites of Davis, the anterior peribulbar sites of Wang or the peri-ocular sites of Weiss and Bloomberg, the medial periconal site of Hustead, sub-Tenon's injection under direct vision or with a cannula as advocated by Greenbaum. Single injection techniques were not devoid of problems. Up to 20% of patients needed additional injections to provide complete akinesia. Optimum insertion sites and safer trajectories of needle paths seemed to be key in providing total akinesia and anaesthesia while keeping the patient and globe safe. Despite these advances, rare but serious complications continued to be reported.

Much controversy existed as to whether it was safer to put dull needles or sharp needles into the orbit or whether the needle should be straight or curved (see 📖 Bevel and gauge, pp. 92–93). Large dull needles can cause more damage to sight and the globe than do fine sharp needles, and the debate continues. The attempts by Straus to use a curved needle with a known radius and short straight segment and Hamilton's custom-bent needle would eventually cause injury as had the curved needle of Siegrist before 1900.

While the new anatomically driven incentive to teaching safer needle techniques was growing, there was a significant change in surgical technique for cataract surgery. Extracapsular cataract surgery was changing to small incision phacoemulsification and implantation of small profile and foldable lenses. Many surgeons were beginning to feel that the marked hypotony produced by ocular compression was unnecessary for less invasive cataract surgical techniques. In fact, some considered it a hindrance for phacoemulsification.

Fichman and Fine reported good results using topical anaesthesia without akinesia during phacoemulsification (see 📖 Timeline, p. 124). Many surgeons avidly encouraged topical anaesthesia and others encouraged sub-Tenon's injection with a blunt cannula (see 📖 Advantages of sub-Tenon's block, p. 115). Unfortunately, topical alone is not applicable to all patients needing eye surgery and the need for safer use of needles or blunt cannulae in the orbit continues.

General anaesthesia

General anaesthesia

General anaesthesia (GA) was introduced in 1846 and became popular with patients because it was an improvement over restraints, alcohol, opium, or mesmeric trance (see Figure 1.1). However, the ophthalmologist did not welcome GA because orbital congestion made the operation more difficult and added to the duration of surgery (see Figure 1.2). In addition, the physical proximity of the anaesthetist, trying to keep the patient breathing and alive, led to friction. Besides, patients died from anaesthesia.

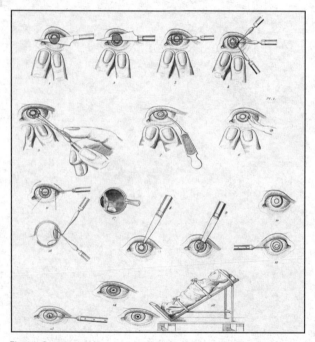

Fig. 1.1 Cataract surgery was quite sophisticated by the mid-nineteenth century. However, prior to the discovery of local and general anesthetics in the latter part of the century, restraints were often employed as means to have patients tolerate eye surgery.

From Carron du Villards, CJF, 1801–1860. Recherches medico-chirurgicales sur l'operation de la cataracte des moyens de la rendre plus sure, et sur l'inutilits des traitments medicaux pour la guerir sans operation. Bruxelles: Societe Typographique Belge, Adolphe Wahlen, 1837, Bascom Palmer Eye Institute's Norton Library collection.

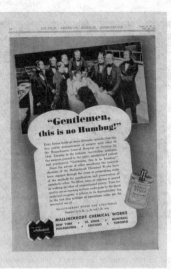

Fig. 1.2 An early advertisement for ether anaesthesia in the Journal of American Medical Association.

From 1846 to 1884 many of the world's ophthalmologists would operate with the patient in restraints, rather than heed their patients' requests for pain relief (see Figure 1.3). After this time, better techniques for maintaining the airway were gradually introduced, but the introduction of improved GA drugs did not follow for some time. In addition, impetus for improvement in GA for eye surgery was slowed greatly by the introduction of cocaine, the first effective topical anaesthetic.

The change from GA to LA was more rapid in the USA; this may have been because there were more trained physician anaesthetists in Europe. GA has become significantly safer and more pleasant with the advent of new drugs to induce and maintain anaesthesia, as well as superb analgesics, muscle relaxants, antiemetics etc. Equally important have been advances in the understanding of physiological control of intra-ocular pressure and monitoring to allow optimal blood gases and cardiovascular control (see 📖 Intra-ocular pressure, pp. 40–43). Advances in the management of the airway, first development of the endotracheal tube (c.1928), intermittent positive pressure ventilation and, more recently, the laryngeal mask airway (1983), have allowed avoidance of the operating field and more physiological conditions within the eye during surgery.

Introduction of vitreoretinal surgery offered a new challenge for GA (see 📖 Practical implications, p. 252). Apart from the often prolonged surgical time, intra-vitreal gas injection demanded that nitrous oxide should not be used as its absorption into the bubble, and subsequent removal when nitrous oxide was discontinued, would affect the volume

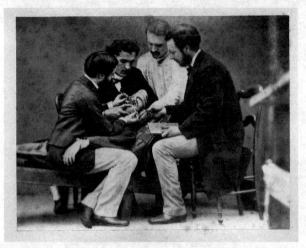

Fig. 1.3 From 1846 to 1884 many of the world's ophthalmologists would operate with the patient actively restrained, rather than heed their patients' requests for pain relief.

From Meyer E, Traite' des Operations, qui se pratiquent sur l'oeil, Treatise of Opertions that are practiced on the eye. Published in Paris in 1871, it was the first textbook of ocular surgery to include photographs and is part of Bascom Palmer Eye Institute's Norton Library collection. Photo by Parisian ophthalmologist, A. de Montmeja, the book's editor and co-author.

of the injected gas and hence the pressure it exerted within the vitreous cavity. In fact, within a few years the use of nitrous oxide as a component of GA declined drastically such that its use must now be rare. For most patients, LA regional orbital blocks provide excellent conditions for VR procedures.

GA has an important place in ophthalmic anaesthesia for children, those patients with learning difficulties and where surgeon or patient have a good reason to request it (see 📖 Indications for general anaesthesia p. 171 & Introduction, p. 186). Contemporary induction agents (e.g. propofol, sevoflurane), avoidance of nitrous oxide, and effective antiemetic drugs (e.g. ondansetron, dexamethasone) have significantly reduced the disadvantages of GA (see 📖 Postoperative complications, p. 372).

Conclusion

Ageing of the population is increasing the demands for ophthalmologic surgery and expectations for a safe, pain-free, and convenient experience. High-volume surgical practices have emerged to meet these demands, which will no doubt lead to further advances in anaesthesia and surgical techniques. Ophthalmic surgical scope extends far beyond cataract surgery and anaesthesia must keep pace with the demands of tumour surgery, retinal relocation and, no doubt, even more sophisticated sight-saving and restoring procedures in the future. The development of GA in ophthalmic surgery occurred before topical and regional anaesthesia. Each area has shown independent progress and only occasionally have developments in one area directly influenced the other. This chapter has summarized highlights of both techniques and related them to the safety of patients and their visual outcome.

Further reading

Atkinson WS. Ophthalmic anaesthesia: the development of ophthalmic anaesthesia. *Am. J. Ophthalmol.* 1961; 51: 1–14.

Calatayud J, Gonzales A. History of the development and evolution of local anesthesia since the coca leaf. *Anesthesiology.* 2003; 98: 1503–08.

Davis II DB, Mandel MR. Peribulbar anaesthesia, a review of technique and complications. *Ophthalmology Clinics of North America.* 1990; 3: 101–9.

Greenbaum S. Parabulbar anesthesia. *Am. J. Ophthalmol.* 1992; 114: 776.

Hustead RF, Hamilton RC in Techniques: Gills JP, Hustead RF, Sanders DR, eds. *Ophthalmic anaesthesia.* Thorofare, NJ: Slack, 1993.

Katsev DA, Drews RC, Rose BT. An anatomic study of retrobulbar needle path length. *Ophthalmology.* 1989; 96: 1221–4.

Knapp H. On cocaine and its use in ophthalmic and general surgery. *Arch. Ophthalmol.* 1884; 13: 402.

Koller K. On the use of cocaine to anaesthetize the eye. As translated by H Knapp in On cocaine and its use in ophthalmic and general surgery. *Arch. Ophthalmol.* 1884; 13: 402–48.

Koornneef L. New insights in the human orbital connective tissue. *Arch. Ophthal.* 1977; 95: 1269–1273.

Local anaesthesia for intraocular surgery. The Royal Colleges of Anaesthetists and Ophthalmologists, UK, 2001.

Van Lint A. Paralysie palpébrale temporarie provoquée dans l'opération de la cataracte. *Ann. Ocul. (Paris)* 1914; 151: 420.

Chapter 2

Anatomic considerations

Dr Jacques Ripart

Introduction

A detailed knowledge of orbital anatomy is essential in order to understand ophthalmic surgery and perform regional orbital anaesthesia safely.

Orbit

The orbit is a cavity in the shape of a truncated square pyramid, with its apex posterior and base corresponding to the anterior aperture.
- The orbital axis is not strictly antero-posterior unlike the visual axis (VA) but is slightly oblique laterally and anteriorly, with an angle of about 30°. Thus, the medial wall of the orbit has a sagittal direction as the lateral wall has a 45° angle (see Figures 2.1a & b).
- The orbital axis is also slightly ascending anteriorly, with the orbital floor being almost horizontal, and the orbital roof has a 30° angle.
- The orbit tends to be close at its frontal aperture, having a C shape rather than a V shape (see Figures 2.2a & 2.2b).
- The orbital rim is oblique laterally and inferiorly. That is why its inferior and lateral angle is located near the equatorial plane of the globe whereas its medial part is located in a plane passing through the anterior pole of the globe (see Figure 2.3).

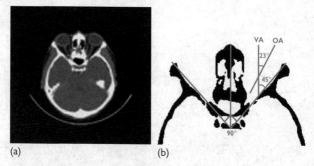

(a)   (b)

Fig. 2.1 (a) Horizontal CT scan of the orbit showings its general shape (pyramid) and orientation. Note that the main orbital axis (OA) is not strictly antero-posteriorly (VA) but slightly oblique laterally, with an angle of about 30° between the visual axis and the orbital axis. (b) Line drawing of the same structures.

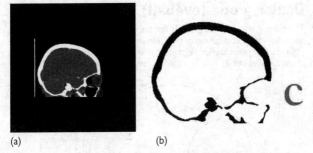

(a)   (b)

Fig. 2.2 (a) Sagittal CT scan of the orbit showing its general shape (pyramid) and orientation. Note that the main orbital axis is not strictly horizontal but slightly upwards and frontwards with an angle of about 30°. Moreover, the orbit tends to be narrower and close to its frontal aperture, (b) having a C shape rather than a V shape.

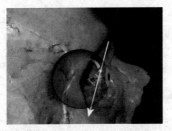

Fig. 2.3 Lateral view of a skull, with a superimposed figurated globe. Note the obliquity of the orbital rim (opening in an inferior and lateral direction). Thus the orbital rim (white arrow) passes through the equator plane near its inferior and lateral angle.

- The average antero-posterior length of the orbit is approximately 40mm. This fact explains why when performing regional anaesthesia with a long needle (e.g. 50mm) it is possible to reach the apex of the orbit, to enter the skull and to inject directly into the cerebrospinal fluid, thus producing total and high spinal anaesthesia.
- The very wide variability in orbit dimensions explains why this complication may occur with the more commonly used needle lengths, e.g. the 35–40mm needles.

Ocular globe (eyeball)

The general shape of the globe is not perfectly spherical. It may be represented by the juxtaposition of two segments of two different spheres (see Figure 2.4). The posterior segment is the main part of the globe. It has a diameter of about 23mm. The anterior segment is the smaller.

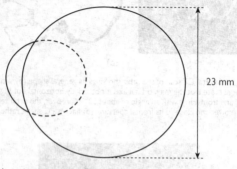

Anterior segment   Posterior segment

Fig. 2.4 schematic view of the general shape of the globe. It is constituted of segments of two spheres with different diameters.

Layers of the globe

The globe is constituted of three layers (see Figure 2.5).
- The outer layer corresponds to the strong and fibrous envelope of the globe and is called the sclerotic coat (sclerotic tissue). The part corresponding to the posterior segment is the sclera that gives to the eyeball its typical white appearance. The part corresponding to the anterior segment is transparent and vessel free and this is called the cornea.

  The junction between sclera and cornea is called the limbus.
- The intermediate layer is called the uvea. In the posterior segment, it is constituted by the vascular layer called the choroid, which provides perfusion to most of the globe. Anteriorly, it continues with the ciliary body that secretes the aqueous humour into the posterior chamber. The iris is a diaphragm that separates the anterior from the posterior chamber. It is inserted peripherally on the ciliary body. The hole located in its centre is the pupil.
- The inner layer is the retina, which is the sensory layer that allows light perception. The emergence of the optic nerve into the globe is called the optic nerve head. On fundoscopy, it is seen as the 'papilla'. Near the posterior pole of the globe, laterally to the papilla, is located the macula which is a part of the retina devoted to central vision, and is vessel-free.

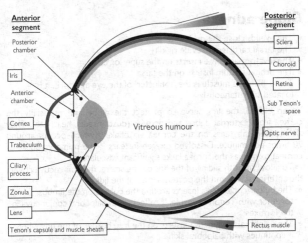

Fig. 2.5 Sagittal schematic view of the globe contents with the insertion of rectus muscles. Note the continuity between the Tenon's capsule and rectus muscles sheaths.

Contents of the globe
- All globe contents are transparent to allow the light to travel to the retina
- The posterior segment is filled with a gel called the vitreous humour
- The anterior segment is filled with the aqueous humour, which is secreted by the ciliary process (part of the ciliary body). It passes through the pupil to reach the anterior chamber where it is resorbed by the trabeculum in the irido-corneal angle, and then evacuated through Schlemm's canal to the episcleral veins
- The anterior and posterior segments are separated by the lens, which is held in place by its ligament, the zonula. The ciliary muscle, by pulling on the zonula, is able to modify the lens curvature, which results in accommodation
- Most of contents of the globe (vitreous humour, lens, aqueous humour) plus the cornea are devoid of any vessels
- Any drugs given systemically will penetrate them poorly
- As a consequence, one must choose specific molecules for intra-ocular penetration (for example fluoroquinolons or fosfomycine for antibiotics) or use very high concentrations (for example sympathicomimetic eye drops to provide iridodilation for surgery)
- Eye drops can flow with the tears through the lacrimal tract, into the nostril, where they can be absorbed by the mucosa and may give rise to clinically noticeable systemic effects

Globe adnexa

- The eyelids close the orbit anteriorly
- The tarsal cartilages provide rigidity
- The levator palpebrae inserts on the superior tarsa
- The orbital septum inserts on the tarsa
- The orbicularis muscle is the 'sphincter' of the eye aperture, it is located subcutaneously

When closed, the lids serve to protect the globe and especially the cornea from external debris and dryness (dust, insects, heat, etc). They also spread the tears on the cornea via blinking which occurs around 20 times per minute. Dissolved oxygen in tears is the primary source of corneal oxygen as the cornea lacks significant vasculature.

To allow smooth sliding of the lids on the sclera, the conjunctiva covers the anterior sclera and the posterior side of the lids.

- The bulbar conjunctiva inserts around the cornea on the limbus together with Tenon's capsule. It reflects with palpebral conjunctiva in the fornixes
- The palpebral conjunctiva inserts on the free border of the lids where it continues with palpebral skin
- The lacrimal gland, located behind the lids in the supero-medial angle, secretes the tears
- Tears drain medially through the lacrimal canals (one inferior and one inferior) and they open on the border of the lids, at the junction between free and lacrimal part of the lids
- The lacrimal canals circle the medial canthus and converge at the lacrimal sac, nasal to the medial canthus
- The lacrimal sac communicates with the nasal fossa (nostril) on the respective side. Here, tears flow to the nose, where they are resorbed by the mucosa

Extra-ocular muscles

There are seven muscles which are of clinical relevance.
- The four rectus muscles of the eye are inserted anteriorly near the equator of the globe
- Posteriorly, they originate together with the levator palpebrae, at the orbital apex, on the tendinous Annulus of Zinn, through which the optic nerve enters the orbit (see Figure 2.6)
- An important property of the extra-ocular muscles is the presence of histologically specific tonic fibres. These fibres respond to an action potential by producing a sustained contraction rather than a single twitch
- This may explain the sustained contractions elicited by suxamethonium that may play a role in increasing the intra-ocular pressure
- The four rectus muscles establish the boundaries of the intramuscular or 'retrobulbar' cone. This cone was once believed to be non-permeable (see Figure 2.7). The intraconal and extraconal spaces are filled with adipose tissues with many areas of communication between the muscles
- The inferior oblique muscle inserts anteriorly near the orbital rim, in the infero-medial angle

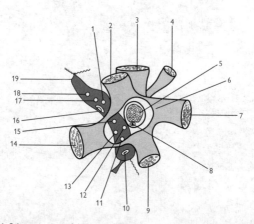

Fig. 2.6 Schematic view of the apex of the orbit, the globe and muscles having been resected. 1, trochlear nerve; 2, superior rectus muscle; 3, levator palpebrae; 4, superior oblique muscle; 5, optic nerve with its meningeal coat; 6, Zinn's annulus; 7, medial rectus muscle; 8, ophthalmic artery; 9, inferior rectus muscle; 10, inferior ophthalmic vein; 11, ocular motor nerve (inferior branch for inferior and medial rectus and inferior oblique muscles); 12, nasociliary nerve; 13, abducens nerve; 14, lateral rectus muscle; 15, ocular motor nerve (superior branch for superior rectus muscle); 16, superior ophthalmic vein; 17, frontal nerve; 18, lacrymal nerve; 19, superior orbital fissure.

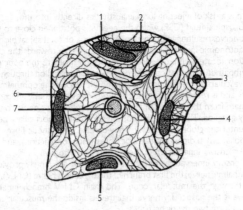

Fig. 2.7 Schematic coronal view of the orbit passing behind the globe. 1, superior rectus muscle; 2, levator palpebrae; 3, superior oblique muscle; 4, medial rectus muscle; 5, inferior rectus muscle; 6, lateral rectus muscle; 7, optic nerve surrounded by its meningeal sheath. Note the complex network of aponeurotic septa that segment the whole adipose corpus of the orbit, without evidence of any inter-muscular membrane.

- Its path is oblique posteriorly and laterally, passing under the inferior rectus muscle
  It then inserts on the sclera, behind the equator, in the infero-lateral quadrant
- The superior oblique muscle originates posteriorly on the Annlus of Zinn
- Its path is first anterior in the angle between the orbital roof and medial wall, outside of the cone, until it forms the trochlea near the supero-medial angle of the orbital rim. It then passes under the superior rectus muscle with a posterior, lateral and inferior direction until its insertion on the sclera, near the posterior pole, in the latero-cephalic quadrant
- The levator palpebrae originates posteriorly on the Annulus of Zinn. Its path follows the superior rectus muscle, just above it
- It passes above the globe and inserts anteriorly on the lid tarsal cartilage
  The lid's orbicularis is a network of subcutaneous fibres forming a sphincter around the lid aperture

Nerve supply of the eye

The optic nerve enters the orbit at its apex through the optic foramen and the Annulus of Zinn (see Figure 2.6).

- Its retrobulbar portion passes through the muscular cone before inserting into the globe
- Embryologically, it is not a cranial nerve (CN) but rather an expansion of the central nervous system. Thus a meningeal sheath, continuous with the cranial meninges, surrounds it

- There is a risk of injecting local anaesthetics directly into the cerebrospinal fluid (CSF) when the needle is positioned close to the optic nerve, resulting in brainstem anaesthesia or total spinal block
- The autonomic innervations of the globe converge towards the ciliary ganglion, located within the muscular cone, cranially to the optic nerve.
- Its sympathetic afferent comes from the stellate ganglion through the peri-vascular plexus (around the carotid). It follows the ophthalmic artery and is responsible for iridodilation. Parasympathetic afferents originate from the nucleus of the CN III and follow this nerve to the ciliary ganglion. The ciliary ganglion then forms the short ciliary nerves that enter the globe posteriorly. They contain sympathetic fibres (iridodilation) and parasympathetic fibres (iridoconstriction), and supply sensory innervation of the iris and ciliary bodies.

The sensory innervations of the globe and orbit are largely provided by the ophthalmic nerve, the first branch of the trigeminal nerve (CN V), which passes through the muscular cone. The main CN V branch innervating the globe is the nasociliary nerve that travels inside the muscular cone. It divides to form two major branches:

- 1: the sensory root of the ciliary ganglion, provides sensory innervations for the iris and ciliary body. Those sensory fibres then travel through the short ciliary nerves until they penetrate the globe
- 2: the long ciliary nerves provide sensory innervations to the main part of the globe

The sensory innervations of the orbit and lids are provided by the frontal nerve (forehead, upper lid and conjunctiva)

- It has an extraconal path, by the terminal branches of the naso-ciliary nerve (medial canthus) and by the infra-orbitary nerve (inferior lid), originating from the maxillary nerve, the second branch of CN penetrating, through the orbital floor
- The trochlear nerve (CN IV) provides the motor supply to the superior oblique muscle
- The abducens nerve (CN VI) supplies the motor supply to the lateral rectus muscle
- The oculomotor nerve (CN III) provides the motor supply to all of the following extra-ocular muscles:
  - Inferior rectus
  - Superior rectus
  - Medial rectus
  - Inferior oblique
  - Levator palpebrae

All the above nerves (except the trochlear nerve) enter the orbit through the greater optic and Annulus of Zinn and then pass through the muscular cone.

Only the motor supply of the orbicularis muscle of the eyelids has an extra-orbital course, coming from the superior branch of the facial nerve (CN VII).

Vascular supply of the orbit

The arterial blood supply of the entire orbit comes from the ophthalmic artery, a branch arising intracranially from the internal carotid artery. It enters the orbit at the apex from the supero-medial side then proceeds through the optic canal and the Annulus of Zinn.

- *There are key anaesthesia ramifications* resulting from the artery's entry into the orbit at this point. Since it enters supero-medially and branches early, the majority of the vasculature travels through the superior aspect of the orbit, rendering the upper half of the orbit more prone to needle-induced trauma
- *Through its course, the artery remains close to* the optic nerve, circling it laterally and anteriorly. Its path is then anterior, cranial and medial

Key branches of the ophthalmic artery include the central retinal artery, and the ciliary arteries that supply the globe. Two-thirds of the retinal blood supply is provided by the choroidal plexus, and one-third from the retinal arteries, which are branches of the central retinal artery.

The orbital veins are located primarily outside of the intramuscular cone. They leave the orbit through the superior orbital fissure en route to the cavernous sinus (see Figure 2.6).

Tenon's capsule

Tenon's capsule is the facial sheath of the eyeball.
- It is a fibroelastic layer that surrounds the entire scleral portion of the globe (see Figures 2.5 and 2.8)
- It defines the episcleral (or sub-Tenon's) space, a potential space with no actual volume, although fluid can be injected into it. Some authors call it the 'articular capsule of the globe'
- Near the equator, Tenon's capsule is perforated by the tendons of the oblique and rectus muscles before they insert into the sclera
- At this point there is continuity between Tenon's capsule and the fascial sheath of these muscles
- Anteriorly, Tenon's capsule fuses with the bulbar conjunctiva before both insert onto the corneal limbus
- Injecting a high volume of fluid (i.e. more than 5cc) into the sub-Tenon's space is therefore likely to cause chemosis (swelling of conjunctiva)

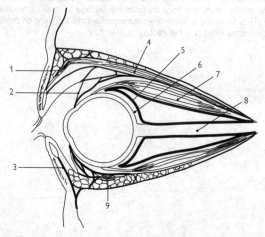

Fig. 2.8 Tenon's apparatus. Schematic sagittal view of the orbit. 1 and 3, orbital septum; 2, bulbar conjunctiva; 4, levator palpebrae muscle; 5, Tenon's capsule (fascial sheath of the eyeball); 6, episcleral space (sub-Tenon's space); 7, superior rectus muscle with its sheath continuing the Tenon's capsule; 8, optic nerve with its meningeal coat; 9, inferior oblique muscle.

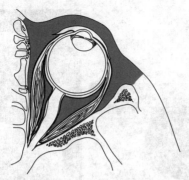

Fig. 2.10 Retro-peribulbar space. Schematic horizontal view of the orbit. The grey area represents the possible spreading of a local anaesthetic injected into either the retrobulbar or peribulbar spaces.

Sub-Tenon's space

LA injected into the sub-Tenon's space will initially fill the space surrounding the globe. Sensory blockade of the globe is achieved due to the fact that all ciliary nerves pass through this space before entering the globe.

Additionally, if a higher volume is injected (more than 3–5cc), the LA will spread into the muscular sheaths that communicate with the sub-Tenon's space, thus accounting for blockade of the extra-ocular muscles and globe akinesia.

Excess fluid will flow under the conjunctiva, which fuses with Tenon's capsule anteriorly (see Figures 2.11a, 2.11b and 2.12). This explains why chemosis is almost universal after a large volume sub-Tenon's injection, a predictable side effect more than a complication.

Finally, as Tenon's capsule is not necessarily completely sealed anteriorly excess of LA may flow toward the lids, causing orbicularis muscle blockade.

Another explanation of the pathogenesis of sub-Tenon's anaesthesia has been postulated. Local anaesthetics may flow towards the muscular cone through the Tenon's capsule, which is not sealed near the posterior pole. Ultrasounds imaging demonstrates that LA is not retained longer than for 2min in the sub-Tenon's space.

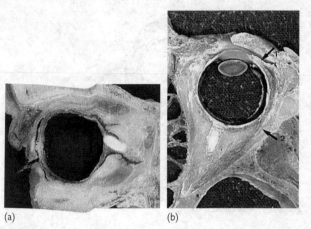

(a)   (b)

Fig. 2.11 Injection of a blue dye into the sub-Tenon's space. (a) Transverse view and sagittal view (bottom). Note the spreading in the sub-Tenon's space, in the medial rectus muscle sheath (2), into the lids, and finally into the cone.

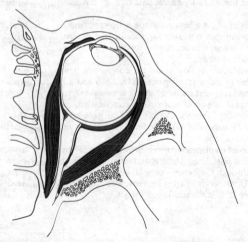

Fig. 2.12 Sub-Tenon space injection (schematic horizontal view of the orbit). The grey area represents possible spreading of any fluid injected into the Tenon's space. Note the selective spreading toward the rectus muscles sheaths, under the conjunctiva, and into the lids.

Conclusion

A detailed knowledge of orbital anatomy is essential in order to understand ophthalmic surgery and to perform RA safely.

Further reading

Dutton JJ. *Atlas of clinical and surgical orbital anatomy*. Philadelphia: W.B. Saunders Co. Ltd, 1994.

Snell RS, Lemp MA. *Clinical anatomy of the eye*. Oxford: Blackwell Scientific Publications, 1989.

Standring S, Ellis H, Healy J, Johnson D, Williams A. *Gray's anatomy: The anatomical basis of clinical practice*, 40th edn. Edinburgh: Churchill Livingston, 2008.

Chapter 3

Ocular physiology relevant to ophthalmic anaesthesia

Dr Anjolie Chhabra

Introduction

The eye is a highly complex organ responsible for the sense of sight. In order to accurately perform this function the eye has many specialized parts and a complex physiology.

Intra-ocular pressure

Intra-ocular pressure (IOP) normally varies from 10–21mmHg. Diurnal variations in IOP in the range of 4–6mmHg are considered normal, as are similar fluctuations with changes in body position or transient increases during coughing and straining.

The IOP is determined by a careful balance of:

- Aqueous humour dynamics
- Volume of the other fluid contents (vitreous and choroidal blood) of the eye
- Scleral rigidity
- External forces acting on the eye such as extraocular muscle tone
- A precipitous increase in IOP can be detrimental in patients with penetrating/perforating eye injuries or those with raised IOP undergoing intra-ocular surgery
- A sudden increase in IOP in these situations can result in vitreous prolapse or even expulsive haemorrhage
- Control of IOP during ophthalmic anaesthesia is of the utmost importance and a basic understanding of the aqueous humour dynamics is essential

Aqueous humour (fluid) dynamics

- Aqueous humour is the clear watery fluid produced by the ciliary body in the posterior chamber of the eye
- It is a complex mixture of electrolytes, organic solutes, growth factors, and other proteins that provide nutrition to the lens, cornea, and other avascular structures in the anterior segment of the eye
- The aqueous humour circulates from the ciliary body, around the iris, through the pupil into the anterior chamber of the eye and exits the globe via two distinct pathways (see Figure 3.1)
- The conventional outflow of aqueous humour is through the angle formed by the cornea and peripheral border of the iris to:
  - The trabecular meshwork (the site of maximum resistance to outflow)
  - Onward to the canals of Schlemm
  - Then drainage into the episcleral veins, the cavernous sinus and finally into the jugular veins
- The secondary route is uveoscleral
  - This accounts for variable aqueous outflow
  - The aqueous humour penetrates the ciliary muscle and then exits through the supraciliary space into the emissarial canals and the choroidal vessels
  - Drainage through this route decreases with increasing age such that the conventional pathway has to compensate to maintain normal IOP.
- Aqueous humour formation is independent of changes in IOP
- Therefore, any factor decreasing the outflow of aqueous humour can cause the IOP to rise
- A combination of factors may determine acute changes in IOP, so correlation with the clinical situation is essential

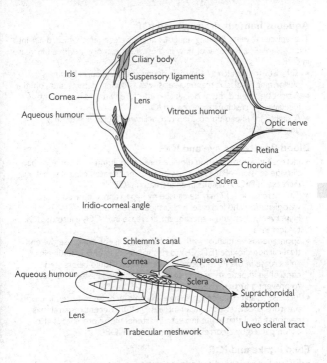

Aqueous outflow

Fig. 3.1 Schematic diagram to show aqueous flow and circulation.

Perioperative factors which affect IOP

- External pressure on the eye
- Increased tone of orbicularis oculi muscle—forceful squeezing of the eyelid can increase IOP up to 70–80mmHg
- Applying an eye speculum can increase IOP by 4–5mmHg
- Needle-based blocks can cause the IOP to rise. The return of the IOP to baseline can take 5–10min with or without the application of an external compression device
- Sustained compression with an external compression device (Honan's balloon or 'super pinky') applied to a relaxed eye for 10–20min can decrease the IOP to below baseline values for as long as 20–25min. Less than 25mmHg pressure should be applied as excessive external pressure can hamper perfusion of the eye as it is mainly composed of water (90%)

Aqueous humour drainage and IOP

The episcleral veins draining aqueous are valveless veins which drain into the jugular veins. Reversal of flow in these veins can occur with an increase in CVP.

- IOP rises to as much as 40mmHg during coughing, bucking, during performing a Valsalva manoeuvre as well as during retching and vomiting
- A tight tie around the neck can also interfere with drainage of the jugular veins resulting in increased IOP
- A slight (15°) head-up position can facilitate jugular vein drainage and decrease IOP

Blood flow to the eye and IOP

- Increase in arterial carbon dioxide tension (pulmonary arterial carbon dioxide tension—$PaCO_2$): it has been demonstrated clinically that an increase in $PaCO_2$ results in an increase in IOP
- The increase in IOP may be caused by hypercapnia-induced vasodilatation and increase in choroidal blood volume
- Hyperventilation and a subsequent decrease in $PaCO_2$ cause the IOP to decrease
- Spontaneous ventilation with an inhalational agent can cause the end tidal carbon dioxide ($ETCO_2$) to rise to 50–55 mmHg resulting in an increase in the IOP. Therefore, ventilation should be assisted or controlled in patients with raised IOP undergoing intra-ocular surgery to prevent a further rise
- Increase in arterial blood pressure: chronic increase in systemic blood pressure is associated with an increase in IOP. Recent research has demonstrated that acute increase in arterial blood pressure is also accompanied by a corresponding increase in IOP

Fluid intake and IOP

- Fasting for prolonged periods can result in a decrease in IOP. Similarly an excessive amount of oral or intravenous fluid can affect IOP as seen in fluid-overloaded burns patients or following haemodialysis when there is a decrease in the serum osmolarity
- Hyperosmotic agent like mannitol decreases IOP by producing osmotic diuresis and probably decreasing vitreous volume. The effect starts 30min after administration of the mannitol and returns to baseline after 2h

Position and IOP

- IOP has been found to be higher in patients positioned prone or in Trendelenburg's position for a prolonged period. The cause of the raised IOP is thought to be a combination of increased episcleral venous pressure combined with an increase in $ETCO_2$ and fluid overload

Anaesthetic drugs and IOP

- Most intravenous induction agents, i.e. barbiturates, benzodiazepines and propofol, cause a decrease in IOP
- Ketamine is controversial. It may increase IOP; however, the effect may be less pronounced at lower doses (1–2mg/kg IV) and in combination with agents which lower IOP it may help to keep IOP closer to pre-induction values
- All inhalational agents including sevoflurane and desflurane decrease IOP

- Non-depolarizing muscle relaxants do not alter IOP
- Premedication with dexmedetomidine or gabapentin decreases IOP

Suxamethonium (succinylcholine) administration and IOP

- May result in an increase in IOP which peaks 90s after administration and can last for 3–6min. This increase in IOP is thought to be due to tonic contractions of extra-ocular muscle fibres. However, an increase in IOP has been observed even in enucleated eyes and a combination of increase in central venous pressure (CVP), choroidal blood flow and cycloplegic effect of suxamethonium have been postulated to be responsible
- The increase in IOP caused by suxamethonium has previously been considered to be deleterious with perforating eye injuries where extrusion of vitreous and eye contents can occur through the wound with an increase in IOP
- However, there are no case reports in the literature to support this belief
- Patients with perforating eye injuries may be 'full stomach' patients who require rapid sequence induction with either suxamethonium or rocuronium to secure the airway
- Before proceeding with the surgery it is imperative to ascertain from the ophthalmologist whether the injured eye is viable
- In addition it is important to assess the patient's airway to determine if difficulty with ventilation or intubation may be encountered
- If the eye is viable and the patient has an anticipated difficult intubation, suxamethonium because of its shorter duration of action as compared to rocuronium can be a safer choice
- In case ventilation and intubation are not anticipated to be difficult and the injured eye is viable, rocuronium can be used instead of suxamethonium for rapid sequence intubation as it provides comparable intubating conditions without producing an increase in IOP
- Laryngoscopy and induction and intubation have been found to cause a greater increase in IOP than that observed after suxamethonium administration
- Therefore, ensuring an adequate depth of anaesthesia is essential, as intubating in a light plane can result in sympathetic stimulation and a precipitous increase in IOP
- Increase in IOP with suxamethonium and intubation can be attenuated by barbiturate (thiopentone) or propofol prior to administering suxamethonium or pre-treatment with short-acting opioids (remifentanil, alfentanil, sufentanil, fentanyl). Administration of intravenous lignocaine 1.5mg/kg at least 90s prior to intubation is known to help. Clonidine along with alfentanil, glyceryl trinitrate (GTN) and nifedepine have all been found to attenuate the increase in IOP

Effects of laryngeal mask airway and endotracheal intubation and IOP

- Use of a laryngeal mask airway (LMA) instead of direct laryngoscopy and endotracheal intubation during induction of GA offers the distinct advantage of having minimal effect upon IOP
- During emergence from anaesthesia, the LMA is associated with far less airway irritation, so precipitous spikes in IOP associated with coughing or bucking are far less likely at the time of extubation
- Glaucoma patients may have more pronounced increases in IOP with laryngoscopy and intubation, so LMA may confer some advantage

Oculo-cardiac reflex

The oculo-cardiac reflex (OCR) is a trigemino-vagal reflex arc. Stimulation of the sensory branches of the trigeminal nerve anywhere along its intracranial or extracranial course leads to parasympathetic stimulation. This can manifest as bradycardia, junctional rhythms, asystole, hypotension, hypoventilation or gastric hypermotility (see Figure 3.2).

OCR has been defined as either a 10% or 20% decrease in heart rate, junctional rhythms, asystole with or without hypotension observed with traction on the extra-ocular muscles to pressure on the globe encountered during strabismus surgery, retinal detachment repair or enucleation of the eyeball.

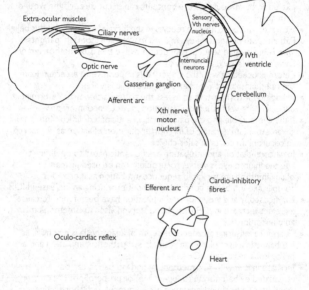

Fig. 3.2 The oculo-cardiac reflex arc.

Neuronal pathway of OCR—afferent arc

Stretch receptors in the extra-ocular muscles are innervated by the sensory fibres of the long and short ciliary nerves which carry impulses via the ciliary ganglion to the Gasserian ganglion and from there onward to the main trigeminal sensory nucleus in the floor of the 4th (IVth) ventricle. Short internuncial fibres in the reticular formation connect the trigeminal nucleus with the motor nucleus of the vagus nerve.

Neuronal pathway of OCR—efferent arc

Inhibitory fibres arising from the motor nucleus of the vagus nerve stimulate the muscarinic receptors in the heart resulting in negative chronotropic or dromotropic effects (conduction).

Facts about OCR

- OCR is more common in children compared to adults
- The incidence of OCR may be higher with medial rectus and inferior oblique manipulation as compared to traction on the lateral rectus muscle
- Adjustment of sutures postoperatively in adjustable suture strabismus surgery may elicit an OCR in awake patients
- The greater the force applied on the muscle, the higher the incidence of OCR and lesser the time taken to achieve a minimum heart rate. Therefore, gentle traction should be applied by the surgeon
- Incidence is minimized following an ophthalmic regional anaesthetic block. Paradoxically, the OCR can be precipitated by the process of instilling the block
- Instillation of topical lignocaine or proxymetacaine decreases the incidence of OCR
- Maintaining an adequate depth of anaesthesia results in a lower incidence of OCR
- Continuous intraoperative monitoring of heart rate, ECG and blood pressure should be done to enable detection of OCR during general anaesthesia
- Arrhythmias observed during an OCR are alarming but they are usually easy to treat and not fatal unless associated with heart disease

Anaesthetic agents and OCR

- Agents with vagomimetic potential are more likely to be associated with OCR
- Propofol-based total intravenous anaesthesia, halothane as compared to isoflurane, sevoflurane or desflurane are associated with a high incidence of OCR
- Opioids like remifentanil, alfentanil or sufentanil are associated with a high incidence of OCR
- Rocuronium and pancuronium are less likely to be associated with OCR because of their vagolytic effects as compared to vecuronium
- Prophylactic administration of anticholinergics can significantly decrease the incidence of OCR but not totally eliminate it
- Intravenous anticholinergics given at the time of induction may be more effective than those administered intramuscularly 30min prior to the surgery
- Intravenous glycopyrrolate may be as effective as atropine in preventing OCR and is associated with lesser tachycardia and incidence of arrhythmias (nodal rhythms and ventricular extrasystoles)

Management of OCR

- Coordination between the surgeon and anaesthetist is essential for management of OCR
- If an OCR is elicited during extra-ocular eye muscle traction the surgeon should be informed and asked to release the muscle
- Gentle traction can be reapplied once the heart rate has returned to baseline
- If the OCR recurs or is very severe, anticholinergics can be administered

Structure and function of globe components

Sclera

The sclera is the outermost opaque fibro-elastic covering of the eye which helps to maintain the shape of the eye. The stroma of the sclera is made up of interlacing collagen fibres of various types and diameters, and complex molecules called proteoglycans. The proteoglycans determine hydration and solute movement through the sclera. They increase in concentration from birth up to the fourth decade and decrease thereafter resulting in decreased elasticity of the sclera. The sclera is less rigid and more prone to collapse in infants and young children. Therefore, whenever large corneo-scleral incisions have to be made in this age group, e.g. for penetrating keratoplasty, scleral support rings such as McNeill Goldman or Flieringa rings of appropriate sizes should be applied.

Cornea

The cornea is the anterior transparent continuation of the sclera. It is composed of three main layers: the corneal epithelium, the substantia propria, and the Descmet's membrane with the underlying endothelium. The epithelial cells of the cornea have remarkable regenerative properties and re-epithelialization of small corneal wounds can occur in 24h, however, damage to the basal layer of the epithelium or the Bowman's membrane can lead to scarring and loss of transparency of the cornea. The substantia propria of the cornea is transparent because collagen fibrils of uniform diameter are arranged in regular hexagonal bundles with uniform interfi-brillar spacing so that light falling on the cornea is uniformly refracted as it enters the eye. As the cornea is avascular it is largely dependent on the aqueous humour bathing its inner surface for its nutrition. The endothelial cells underlying the Descmet's membrane are metabolically active and maintain stromal hydration and transparency by actively removing electrolytes and allowing passive diffusion of water. These cells are of a fixed number and decrease with increasing age and the remaining cells enlarge to compensate for the loss. These cells are sensitive to damage by acids or alkalis but animal experiments and clinical evidence have failed to demonstrate endothelial cell damage with the use of topical local anaesthetics in the eye.

A tear film containing antibacterial lysosomes constantly bathes the cornea, keeping it moist and allowing oxygen to diffuse from the atmosphere to the epithelial cells. A rich supply of sensory nerve fibres from the trigeminal nerve makes the cornea sensitive to injury by dust or foreign bodies. Humans involuntarily blink their lids every 4–6s to moisten the cornea with tears and remove debris. These protective mechanisms are lost in patients under anaesthesia, therefore, to prevent corneal drying and ulceration, the non-operative eye should be taped shut and the eye to be operated irrigated with normal saline. Patients wearing contact lenses should be instructed to remove them prior to anaesthesia as they can interfere with epithelial oxygenation.

Uvea and the choroid

The uveal tract lines the inner surface of the sclera and is composed of the choroid, the ciliary body and the iris. The choroid lies between the sclera and the retina, it is highly vascular and is mainly concerned with the nutrition of the adjacent layers. The ciliary body has two main parts. The anterior part is thrown into folds and is called the pars plicata. Aqueous humour is secreted by the epithelial cells of this part of the ciliary body. Pars plana or the posterior part of the ciliary body is mainly composed of the ciliary muscle. Contraction of these smooth muscle fibres results in decreased tension in the suspensory ligament and an increase in the convexity of the crystalline lens during accommodating for near vision. The ciliary muscle also influences the shape of the trabecular meshwork and regulates the outflow of aqueous humour through the meshwork and the adjoining Schlemm's canal.

The iris is the coloured part of the eye visible through the cornea. It is a diaphragm in the coronal plane suspended from the base of the ciliary body. It has an aperture in the centre called the pupil. In addition to stroma and pigmented epithelium, the iris has a circular band of muscle fibres encircling the pupil called the sphincter pupillae (innervated by postganglionic parasympathetic fibres) and radial muscle fibres called dilator pupillae (supplied by the postganglionic sympathetic fibres).

Pupillary reflex

A sudden bright light falling on the pupil causes it to constrict, whereas when the ambient light is dim the pupils dilate to increase the light entering the eye by as much as 16-fold. This reflex is known as the pupillary reflex.

Neuronal pathway causing pupillary constriction

Some of the neurons transmitting light impulses from the retina leave the optic tract before reaching the lateral geniculate body and terminate in the pretectal nucleus in the midbrain. From here neurons project to the ipsilateral and contralateral Edinger–Westphal nucleii. Neurons originating from the Edinger–Westphal nucleii pass to the ciliary ganglion and the postganglionic parasympathetic fibres reach the iris and ciliary body in both eyes causing ipsilateral as well as contralateral pupillary constriction (consensual light reflex). The fibres synapsing in the pretectal nucleus leave the optic neurons before reaching the lateral geniculate body, therefore at times the pupillary reflex is preserved even when vision is lost (Argyll–Robertson pupil).

Pathway for pupillary dilatation

The centre for pupillary dilatation is situated in the hypothalamus; fibres originating from here descend in the cervical sympathetic chain, synapse in the superior cervical ganglion and reach the iris and ciliary muscles via the long ciliary nerves causing the pupil to dilate when the ambient light decreases.

Retina

The retina is the innermost photosensitive lining of the eye and is made up of ten layers. The layer adjacent to the choroid is the pigment epithelium. The next layer contains the rods (receptors for the monochromatic vision) and cones (receptors for the colour vision). Projecting inwards from these receptors are the neural elements, i.e. the bipolar cells, the ganglion, and the amacrine cells. The axons of these cells join to form the optic nerve which leaves the globe just medial to the posterior pole. As there are no receptors present in this area of the retina is called the 'blind spot'. It is also referred to as the optic disc or optic nerve head.

Examination of the optic disc by an ophthalmoscope can help to diagnose various disease processes, e.g. cupping of the disc in glaucoma, papilloedema or optic disc oedema in patients with raised intracranial pressure. As this is the only area in the body where arteries, arterioles and veins can be seen, ophthalmoscopic examination can ascertain end organ damage in systemic diseases like diabetes and hypertension. Temporal to the optic disc on the retina is a yellowish spot called the fovea centralis which has cones packed tightly together with each synapsing to a bipolar cell. This area of the retina has maximum visual acuity and the eyes move so that images are focused on the fovea.

Extra-ocular muscles

The movements of the eye are controlled by six extra-ocular muscles. The medial and lacteral rectii adduct and abduct the eye. The medially rotated eye is turned upwards by the inferior oblique and downwards by the superior oblique. The laterally rotated eye is turned upwards and downwards by the superior and inferior rectii respectively. The occulomotor nerve supplies the superior, medial, inferior rectus, and inferior oblique. The lateral rectus is supplied by the abducens nerve and the superior oblique by the trochlear nerve. Coordination of both eye movements is essential to prevent diplopia and facilitate binocular vision. This is mediated by the fibres from the lateral geniculate body which in addition to synapsing in the pretectal region of the midbrain also project to the frontal cortex which refines and coordinates extra-ocular eye movements.

Under deep anaesthesia pupils are central and fixed. If at the start of surgery eyes become dysconjugate, i.e. roll up (Bell's phenomenon), or roll down, the plane of anaesthesia is inadequate and this can interfere with the eye surgery. The eye can be made central either by increasing the inspired concentration of the inhalational agent or by administering appropriate muscle relaxants.

Visual pathways

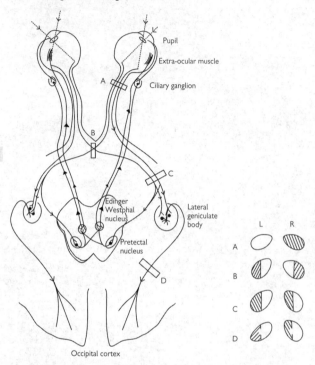

Fig. 3.3 Lesions of the optic nerve marked at various sections as A, B, C, and D.

The impulses generated in the photoreceptors of the retina are transmitted by the bipolar cells (1st-order neurons) to the ganglion cells (2nd-order neurons). A lesion in the optic nerve of one side causes blindness in that eye (see Figure 3.3 lesion A). The axons of the ganglion cells terminate in the lateral geniculate body in the thalamus. Prior to reaching the lateral geniculate body, neurons arising from the nasal half of each retina cross over at the optic chiasma. This accounts for the loss of vision from the opposite sides of both visual fields in case a lesion occurs at the level of the optic chiasma (heteronymous hemianopia, see Figure 3.3 lesion B).

The optic tract distal to the optic chiasma contains the ipsilateral temporal neurons and contralateral nasal neurons. Therefore a lesion in the optic tract distal to the chiasma results in loss of visual field of the same side of both eyes (homonymous hemianopia, see Figure 3.3 lesion C).

From the lateral geniculate body, the third-order neurons pass to the visual cortex also known as the Broadman's area V1. A lesion at the level of the occipital cortex results in discrete visual field defects depending on the area of the cortex affected; macular vision is usually spared because of its large representation in the occipital cortex (see Figure 3.3 lesion D).

Conclusion

Understanding the complex physiology of the eye and its components enables safe and efficient management of patients undergoing anaesthesia for ophthalmic surgery.

Further reading

Arasho B, Sandu N, Spiriev T et al. Management of the trigeminocardiac reflex: facts and own experience. Neurol. India. 2009; 57: 375–80.

Barrett KE, Barman SM, Boitano S, Brooks HL. Vision. In Barrett KE, Barman SM, Boitano S, Brooks HL eds. Ganong's review of medical physiology, 23rd edn. New Delhi: Tata McGraw Hill, 2010: 181–201.

Castejon H, Chiquet C, Savy O et al. Effect of acute increase in blood pressure on intraocular pressure in pigs and humans. Invest. Ophthalmol. Vis. Sci. 2010; 51: 1599–605.

Cheng MA, Todorov A, Tempelhoff R et al. The effect of prone positioning on intraocular pressure in anesthetized patients. Anesthesiology. 2001; 95: 1351–5.

Fautsch MP, Johnson DH. Aqueous humor outflow: what do we know? Where will it lead us? Invest Ophthalmol. Vis. Sci. 2006; 47: 4181–7.

Kelly RE, Dinner M, Turner LS et al. Succinylcholine increases intraocular pressure in the human eye with the extraocular muscles detached. Anesthesiology. 1993; 79: 948–52.

Miller SJ. Anatomy and physiology. In SJ Miller, ed., Parsons' diseases of the eye, 18th edn. Edinburgh: Churchill Livingstone, 1990; 3–23.

Rada JA, Achen VR, Penugonda S et al. Proteoglycan composition in the human sclera during growth and aging. Invest. Ophthalmol. Vis. Sci. 2000; 41: 1639–48.

Smith GB. The physiology of the eye of interest to ophthalmic anaesthetists. In GB Smith, RC Hamilton, CA Carr, eds, Ophthalmic anaesthesia, 2nd edn. London: Hodder Arnold, 1996: 49–56.

Vachon CA, Warner DO, Bacon DR. Succinylcholine and the open globe. Anesthesiology. 2003; 99: 221–3.

Chapter 4

Pharmacology for ophthalmic local anaesthesia

Dr Hamish McLure

Introduction

In the early 1990s, ophthalmic LA was provided almost exclusively by surgeons. Serious complications were known to occur but the surgeons rarely possessed the up-to-date knowledge and skills to manage these sometimes life-threatening events.

In 1993, the Royal College of Anaesthetists and Royal College of Ophthalmologists jointly published guidelines *Local anaesthesia for intra-ocular surgery*. This document described the serious complications that could follow ophthalmic blocks and laid down a framework for providing a safer service. This included a significant role for the anaesthetist in the capacity of anaesthesia provider and lead for resuscitation. Safety was further enhanced by the evolving less invasive techniques of ophthalmic anaesthesia.

Despite the safer environment, significant adverse events can still occur and the LA agents themselves may still be a cause of iatrogenic injury.

For all those involved in the delivery of ophthalmic LA, a sound knowledge of LA pharmacology is essential.

Physiology of nerve conduction

Knowledge of nerve conduction physiology is essential to understanding LA pharmacology as LAs act by inhibiting normal nerve conduction.

The resting membrane potential of a neuron is maintained by a Na/K ATPase pump. It moves three sodium ions from inside to outside the cell in exchange for two potassium ions moving in the opposite direction. The cell membrane is relatively impermeable to sodium but permeable to potassium, which slowly moves down its concentration gradient from inside to outside the cell. This combination of the active removal of positively charged sodium ions and the passive movement of positively charged potassium ions from inside to outside the cell, produces a trans-membrane resting potential of −70 millivotls (mV) (inside negative compared to outside). A brief reversal of the normal resting membrane potential, caused by an altered distribution of ions, is called an action potential. Conduction of nerve impulses occurs through propagation of action potentials down an axon. Stimulation of a nerve results in opening of membrane sodium channels, causing an influx of sodium ions and a local area of depolarization. If this local depolarization is large enough to reach a threshold potential (−60mV) then an action potential is generated. Large numbers of voltage-sensitive sodium channels open and the resulting influx of sodium ions cause a sudden rise in the transmembrane potential to +30mV, after which the sodium channels close. Potassium efflux and the continued action of Na/K ATPase restore the original ion concentration gradients and resting membrane potential. The sodium channels have a brief refractory period during which they are unable to re-open, preventing retrograde transmission and ensuring only 'forward' propagation down the axon.

LA agents act by reversibly blocking voltage gated sodium channels in the neuron (or other excitable tissue) cell membrane. As the LA can only block the channel from inside the cell it must first traverse the cell membrane. By blocking the voltage-gated sodium channels, LAs prevent generation and propagation of action potentials and therefore halt the sensory, motor or autonomic function of the neuron. LA agents do not alter either the resting membrane potential or the threshold potential.

Pharmacology of local anaesthetic agents

Structure

Local anaesthetics in common usage are either ester or amide compounds. They consist of a lipophilic aromatic ring joined by either an ester or amide linkage to a hydrophilic amine group (see Figure 4.1). Esters are inherently more unstable than amides and tend to have a shorter shelf life.

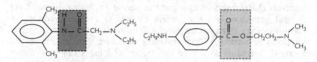

Fig. 4.1 Diagram demonstrating the structure of lidocaine with its amide linkage (left) and tetracaine with its ester bond (right).

Ionization

All LA agents are weak bases and exist in a dynamic equilibrium of ionized and unionized forms.

The pKa of a drug is the pH at which it exists in equal proportions of ionized and unionized states. In a neutral pH environment, local anaesthetics predominantly exist in an ionized state, as their pKa exceeds 7.4. The relationship between the pH, pKa and relative qualities in ionized and unionized states is given by the Henderson–Hasselbach equation:

$$pH = pKa + log\ [unionized]/[ionized]$$

In order to block the sodium channel, and therefore neuronal depolarization, the LA agent must first penetrate the neuronal cell membrane lipid bilayer. Only a unionized drug is lipid-soluble and able to penetrate the membrane, therefore alkali conditions or agents with a lower pKa are associated with shorter onset times. Following entry into the nerve, the more acidic intracellular milieu restores drug to an ionized state which then blocks activated voltage-gated sodium channels. If the drug encounters acidic tissue conditions outside the cell, perhaps as a result of local infection or inflammation, a greater percentage remains ionized and less agent is able to penetrate the cell membrane. Local infection or inflammation often results in ineffectual LA blocks.

Isomerism

Organic compounds that contain a carbon atom linked to four different chemical groups can exist in two conformations that are mirror images of each other. These arrangements are 'stereo-isomers' of the parent compound. Several anaesthetic agents, e.g. bupivacaine and ropivacaine, display stereo-isomerism. The isomers may be differentiated by the direction they rotate polarized light and are labelled either S (–) laevorotatory or R (+) dextrorotatory. The physical properties of stereo-isomers are usually identical, but their *in vivo* characteristics may differ. S (–) bupivacaine (levobupivacaine) has similar LA properties to R (+) bupivacaine, but *in vitro* in animal and volunteer studies it has an improved safety profile over racemic bupivacaine. Ropivacaine is marketed as an enantiopure preparation.

Potency

The potency of a LA is dictated by its lipid solubility. A more lipid-soluble anaesthetic is better able to penetrate the neuron cell membrane and gain access to the sodium channels. Lipid solubility is measured in the laboratory by noting the distribution of agent between adjacent aqueous and non-aqueous solvent (e.g. octanol) phases. This allows calculation of a solvent partition coefficient. The higher the coefficient, the more lipid-soluble and potent the drug. Other factors that may influence the potency of a LA are its vasodilator properties and its tissue distribution, both of which influence mass of drug presenting to the cell membrane.

Duration of action

The duration of action of anaesthetic agents is proportional to its protein binding. LAs can bind to plasma (albumin and α1-acid glycoprotein) and tissue proteins. Albumin is a low-affinity, high-volume site compared to α1-acid glycoprotein which is a high-affinity but relatively low-volume site of binding. Only unbound LA is active. Tissue-bound drug acts as a reservoir and prolongs the duration of action. Changes in the proportion of drug bound to plasma and tissue proteins such as due to a change in pH can precipitate toxicity by a sudden increase in free, unbound drug. Protein binding tends to increase following surgery or trauma and decreases in pregnancy or with use of the contraceptive pill.

Vasodilator properties

Most LA agents at concentrations commonly used in ophthalmic anaesthesia cause vasodilatation. Some drugs may cause vasoconstriction at higher concentrations. Cocaine is the exception as it produces intense vasoconstriction by inhibiting the reuptake of catecholamines.

Metabolism and excretion

Amide LAs are metabolized by amidases in the liver to inactive compounds which are excreted in the urine. Prilocaine is the most rapidly metabolized and bupivacaine is the slowest. Metabolism occurs in two phases: phase I metabolism includes hydroxylation, N-dealkylation and methylation, followed by phase II where the metabolites are conjugated with amino acids into less active and inactive metabolites. The rate of elimination of prilocaine exceeds that possible from hepatic metabolism alone, which may be explained by pulmonary uptake. Extravascular lung tissue has a lower pH which causes ion trapping and sequestration of prilocaine, helping to prevent sudden rises in free unbound plasma levels.

Ester LAs are rapidly metabolized by plasma and tissue cholinesterases. The ubiquitous nature of these enzymes ensures rapid metabolism and a low risk of toxicity. One of the main metabolites of cholinesterases is p-amino benzoic acid (PABA) which has occasionally been associated with allergic reactions. Patients with atypical plasma cholinesterases may be at higher risk of developing toxicity from ester anaesthetics due to slower or absent plasma hydrolysis. Cocaine is again an exception, as it is metabolized by liver hydrolysis with metabolites eliminated in the urine.

Table 4.1 Pharmacological properties of local anaesthetic agents

	Partition coefficient	Potency	pKa	Onset	Protein binding (%)	Duration	Toxic concentration
Cocaine	—	High	8.7	Slow	98	Long	—
Amethocaine	221	Intermediate	8.5	Slow	76	Intermediate	—
Lidocaine	43	Intermediate	7.7	Fast	64	Intermediate	>5mcg/ml
Bupivacaine	346	High	8.1	Intermediate	95	Long	>1.5mcg/ml
Ropivacaine	115	Intermediate	8.2	Intermediate	94	Long	>4mcg/ml
Prilocaine	25	Intermediate	7.8	Fast	55	Intermediate	>5mcg/ml
Articaine	17	Intermediate	7.8	Fast	95	Intermediate	—

Toxicity

Toxicity may be local, central or systemic.

Local

LAs are neurotoxic in high concentration or when nerves are exposed to lower concentrations for a prolonged period. In ophthalmic anaesthesia, standard concentrations of LAs are in contact with nerve tissue for a relatively short period of time. However, LAs might contribute to nerve damage where there is high orbital pressure, low systemic blood pressure or co-existent local vascular disease.

LAs may also be toxic to muscle tissue. Direct injection into the delicate extra-ocular muscles may result in tissue necrosis, scarring, and restricted function. This muscle damage can lead to strabismus requiring surgical correction. The risk of permanent damage is higher with the co-administration of vasoconstrictors, and appears to be lower if the LA mixture contains hyaluronidase.

Central

The optic nerve is surrounded proximally by a dural sheath containing cerebrospinal fluid (CSF). Central toxicity may arise from inadvertent perforation of the dural sheath with injection of LA into the subarachnoid space. The classic symptoms and signs of a total spinal anaesthesia are characterized by rapid loss of consciousness, cardiovascular instability, and respiratory then cardiac arrest. Management is supportive with oxygen and intubation if required, assistance with ventilation and appropriate cardiovascular support.

Systemic

Systemic toxicity is caused by a high plasma concentration of LA and may result from either excessive dosing by an appropriate route or inadvertent intravascular injection. Given the relatively small doses of LA used in ophthalmic block, and the vascularity of the orbit, an intravascular injection is more likely.

The two main sites of excitable tissues in the body are those primarily affected by elevated plasma levels of LAs. Initially central nervous system toxicity gives rise to peri-oral paraesthesia, metallic taste, slurred speech, dizziness, tinnitus, agitation, confusion, and convulsions. At very high plasma concentrations, widespread blockade of sodium channels causes neuron suppression and coma.

Cardiovascular effects usually follow neurological toxicity and initially consist of bradycardia, prolongation of the PR interval and a widened QRS complex. Further rises in plasma levels can cause a spectrum of dysrrthymias including bradycardia, ectopic beats, re-entry tachycardia and eventually ventricular fibrillation.

The management of systemic LA toxicity is largely supportive including cardiopulmonary resuscitation if required. Oxygen, fluids, vasopressors, inotropes, antiarrhythmics, and anticonvulsants may all be required. Infusion of lipid emulsion (e.g. intralipid) is a now a recommended specific therapy for systemic toxicity and acts by binding free unbound LA agent, reversing the concentration gradient between plasma and excitable tissues.

There is evidence for its use in cases of cardiorespiratory arrest and it may also have a role in less severe cases of toxicity.

The risk of systemic (and central) toxicity may be reduced by adopting several 'safety nets' into routine clinical practice: careful needle placement, aspiration prior to every slow injection, fractionated doses, adequate time between doses, the use of a less toxic LA, awareness of maximum safe doses and the addition of other drugs (e.g. hyaluronidase, bicarbonate, epinephrine) to reduce the mass of LA required.

Genuine immune-mediated allergic reactions to amide LA agents are extremely rare. LA agents consist of small molecules that are generally non-antigenic. They may occasionally act as a hapten by binding to plasma proteins and triggering an immune response. Many self-reported incidents of 'allergy' often turn out to be related to epinephrine-containing solutions given partially intravascularly whilst sitting up in the dentist's chair. However, all patients presenting with a clear history suggestive of LA allergy must be appropriately investigated in an immunology clinic.

In contrast, allergy to ester anaesthetics is much more common. It is often due to allergy to PABA, one of the rapidly produced metabolites of ester agents. Patients may become sensitized to PABA either through previous administration of ester anaesthetics or though exposure to preservatives in cosmetic and some foodstuffs which have similar antigenic properties. There is cross-reactivity between sulphonamide compounds and PABA and caution should be applied when using ester agents in patients with a known sulphonamide allergy.

Individual agents

Cocaine

Although no longer used as an anaesthetic agent in ophthalmic surgery, the effects of cocaine on the conjunctiva marked the birth of LA. Cocaine is an ester LA derived from the leaves of the erthroxylan coca plant from Peru. Carl Koller, an ophthalmic surgeon working in Vienna in 1884, discovered the LA properties of cocaine after instilling it into his own eye. Cocaine's career as an ophthalmic anaesthetic was short due to frequent reports of systemic toxicity and death following orbital injection. Cocaine causes tachycardia, hypertension, sweating, nausea and other hyperexcitable side effects when given systemically. Despite this unappealing toxicity profile it continues to be a popular drug of abuse. Cocaine's only remaining common use in clinical medicine is as a component of Moffatt's solution (2mls 8% cocaine, 2mls 1% sodium bicarbonate and 1ml 1:1000 adrenaline) used for nasal mucosa preparation prior to ear nose and throat (ENT) or dacryocystorhinostomy (DCR) surgery.

Tetracaine

Tetracaine or amethocaine is an ester LA. A 0.5–1% solution can be applied topically to the conjunctiva prior to orbital nerve blocks. Its main side effect is that it stings on instillation and is relatively toxic to the cornea. Amethocaine is also available as a 4% cream which produces good topical anaesthesia for venepuncture, venous cannulation or trancutaneous orbital injection.

Oxybuprocaine

Oxybuprocaine is an ester LA with a more favourable side effect profile compared to amethocaine. It is available in a 0.5% solution for ophthalmic use, is less painful on instillation and is less toxic to the cornea.

Proxymetacaine

Proxymetacaine is an alternative ester LA to oxybuprocaine. It is available in a 0.5% solution and is non-irritant even in atopic individuals.

Lidocaine

Lidocaine was one of the earliest of the amide LA agents and is still in common use today. It is a tertiary amide derived from diethylamino-acetic acid. It is moderately potent and has a rapid onset of action. It is 70% protein-bound and when used in ophthalmic blocks has duration of approximately 1 hour. Clinicians' familiarity with the drug and its favourable toxicity profile has ensured that lidocaine remained a popular choice of LA.

Bupivacaine

Bupivacaine was introduced in 1963. It is fourfold as potent as lidocaine and has a longer duration of action. When used for peribulbar anaesthesia as a 0.75% solution, up to 70% of patients may have persistent sensory deficits and diplopia the day after surgery. In the elderly this may prove significantly disabling. Bupivacaine is therefore commonly mixed with lidocaine with the intention of producing a LA solution with rapid onset and long duration. In reality it will have intermediate properties between lidocaine and bupivacaine. Bupivacaine has a pKa of 8.1 and is 95% protein-bound. Systemic toxicity can be severe, requiring prolonged supportive resuscitation.

Levobupivacaine

Levobupivacaine is an enantiopure preparation of S (–) bupivacaine. The S enantiomer of bupivacaine is significantly less toxic in overdose than the racemic mixture. It requires a higher plasma level of levobupivacaine to cause either convulsions or myocardial depression than with racemic bupivacaine. Levobupivacaine is available as 2.5, 5.0 and 7.5mg/ml solutions, with the latter most suited to ophthalmic anaesthesia.

Ropivacaine

Ropivacaine is another enantiopure (S-isomer) preparation of an amide LA related to bupivacaine and mepivacaine. It is manufactured in three concentrations: 2, 7.5 and 10mg/ml. Its main advantage over racemic bupivacaine is a safer toxicity profile. It is also less lipid-soluble than bupivacaine which may explain its apparent motor neuron-sparing effect. Motor block with low concentrations of ropivacaine tends to be slower in onset and of shorter duration than after an equivalent dose of racemic bupivacaine. This subtle effect is not apparent when 0.75% ropivacaine is used for ophthalmic anaesthesia, where a degree of akinesia is often desirable. Ropivacaine has a similar potency to bupivacaine, a pKa of 8.1 and is 94% protein-bound.

Prilocaine

Prilocaine is an amine analogue of lidocaine. Its main advantage over other LA agents is its rapid clearance from plasma and excellent safety record. It is the drug of choice for total intravenous RA. Prilocaine 4% and 3% with felypressin lost their license for ophthalmic anaesthesia in the UK amid concerns about optic nerve and retinal toxicity. The less concentrated 1% and 2% forms may still be used but these are less effective than alternative agents.

A well-known but rarely seen side effect is methaemoglobinaemia. Should the patient become symptomatic, high concentrations of oxygen and intravenous methyl blue should be administered.

Prilocaine and lidocaine as their crystalline bases may be mixed to form EMLA (eutatic mixture of LA). A eutectic mixture is one where two compounds mixed together form a substance with a single set of physical characteristics. The low melting point of this mixture means it can be made into a cream at room temperature. EMLA cream is an alternative to amethocaine for producing cutaneous topical anaesthesia.

Articaine

Articaine is an amide local anaesthetic first used in Germany in the 1970s. It differs from other amide agents in having a thiophene ring and an additional ester linkage. The thiophene ring increases its lipid solubility, which in addition to a low pKa gives it an onset time similar to prilocaine. The additional ester linkage means it is rapidly metabolized by plasma cholinesterases in a similar fashion to ester anaesthetics. This rapid onset and offset profile makes it a useful agent for ophthalmic anaesthesia as prolonged akinesia may be avoided. An alternative agent should be sought in those patients with a history suggestive of atypical cholinesterases.

Additives

Hyaluronidase

Hyaluronidase is an enzyme used to break down hyaluronic acid in the connective tissue which binds cells together. The preparation used in the UK is derived from sheep's testis. Recombinant versions are available in some countries. The potential benefits of adding hyaluronidase to LA mixtures in ophthalmic blocks include increased speed of onset and minimizing increases in orbital pressure by allowing distribution of LA away from the site of injection. The evidence for the effectiveness of hyaluronidase in the clinical setting is conflicting, with some papers suggesting as little as 7.5IU/ml being effective, and other authors detecting no benefit with 150IU/ml. There is consistent evidence of a beneficial effect in sub-Tenon's and retrobulbar anaesthesia, but the data is mixed on peribulbar techniques. If this is examined more closely there appears to be a volume effect. When using higher volumes, hyaluronidase has little impact. Any benefit may be hidden in high-volume peribulbar techniques as there is sufficient volume to reach target nerves without the added effect of hyaluronidase. However, in peribulbar blocks using lower volumes hyaluronidase seems to increase both the speed of onset and quality of the block. Sub-Tenon's and retrobulbar blocks require low volumes of LA and are improved with the addition of hyaluronidase. Side effects are rare but include the formation of orbital pseudotumours and systemic allergic reactions.

Epinephrine

Most LA agents are vasodilators at clinical concentrations. The addition of a vasoconstrictor to LA mixtures for ophthalmic anaesthesia confers the potential advantages of prolonging the duration of action, minimizing the increase in orbital pressure following injection and slowing the rise in systemic plasma levels. The most commonly used vasoconstrictor is epinephrine in a dose of 5mcg/ml (1 in 200,000). This concentration can be made up by adding 0.1ml of 1:1000 epinephrine to 20mls of LA solution. Potential side effects include impairing blood flow to the eye. Doppler studies have confirmed reduced retinal perfusion pressures in primate models when retrobulbar injections include epinephrine. Systemic side effects such as tachycardia and hypertension may also result from intravenous absorption or inadvertent intravenous injection.

Sodium bicarbonate

LA agents are weak bases and exist in ionized and non-ionized forms depending on the pH of their environment. In alkaline conditions, more of the drug exists in an unionized, lipid-soluble state. The addition of sodium bicarbonate to raise the pH of a LA mixture may therefore improve onset times. The potential pitfalls of altering the mixture pH include precipitation of drugs out of solution and the inactivation of other additives, e.g. epinephrine.

Other additives

As with other regional anaesthetic techniques, clinicians have experimented with other additive to improve the effectiveness or duration of blocks. These include muscle relaxants, opiates and α_2 agonists. None have found universal acceptance and care must be taken when preparing increasingly complex drug cocktails to avoid dosing errors or incompatibility problems.

Future agents

Diphenhydramine

Diphenhydramine is a topical antihistamine utilized for it antipruritic effects. Along with selected other antihistamines, it is known to have LA properties. Recent trials of 5% diphenhydramine against saline control in rabbits have demonstrated a rapid onset and relatively short-acting LA profile. It may be useful in patients with corneal disease that need to avoid the potentially toxic effects of ester anaesthetics. It may also prove useful in the small cohort of patients with ester anaesthetic or PABA allergy.

Conclusion

Significant adverse events can occur during ophthalmic anaesthesia and the LA agents themselves may be a cause of iatrogenic injury. For all those involved in the delivery of ophthalmic LA, a sound knowledge of local anaesthetic pharmacology is essential.

Further reading

Kumar C, Dodds C and Fanning G. *Ophthalmic anaesthesia*, 1st edn. Lisse: Swets and Zeitlinger; 2002.
Local anaesthesia for intraocular surgery. Accessed 13 May 2010. http://www.rcoa.ac.uk/docs/ RCARCOGuidelines.pdf.
McLure HA, Rubin AP. Review of local anaesthetic agents. *Minerva Anestesiol.* 2005; 71: 59–74.
Peck TE, Hill SA, Williams M. *Pharmacology for anaesthesia and intensive care*, 2nd edn. London: Greenwich Medical Media; 2004.
Rubin AP. Anaesthesia for cataract surgery – time for a change? *Anaesthesia.* 1990; 45: 717–18.
Suffridge PJ, Wiggins MN, Landes RD, Harper RA. Diphenhydramine as a topical ocular anaesthetic. *Can. J. Ophthalmol.* 2009; 44: 181–4.

Preoperative assessment and preparation

Dr Marc Feldman

Introduction

Preoperative assessment is essential for the formulation of a good anaesthetic management plan. Inadequate preparation preoperatively can result in anaesthetic morbidity and mortality. This is particularly relevant for ophthalmic patients, where the age range varies from premature to elderly, surgery involves routine and emergency which are simple or very complex.

Goals of preoperative assessment

Good care begins with a good preoperative evaluation. Goals of preoperative evaluation include:

- Establishment of a doctor–patient relationship
- Psychological preparation of the patient
- Perioperative risk assessment
- Obtaining informed consent
- Anaesthetic management planning

Preoperative evaluation has additional benefits. General medical screening can be good preventive medicine. This can lead to earlier treatment for newfound conditions. Overall medical care can be improved for known conditions which have not yet been optimized. The preoperative assessment is an opportunity not only to modify operative risk, but also to address long-term health issues. The preoperative assessment can be an opportunity to educate and motivate for smoking cessation, exercise, and dietary management. Some patients will be found sufficiently ill in the preoperative clinic to need emergency admission to the hospital.

Preoperative evaluation can have potential problems as well. Rapport between physicians can be strained as differences of opinion on management arise. There can be inconsistencies in care. This can lead to inefficiencies, confusion, and frustration to the patient and the medical care team. Last-minute cancellation of surgery for preoperative issues leads to disruption of the operating room schedule.

Doctor–patient relationship

Eye surgery is the most common surgical procedure in the elderly. In the US, the Medicare programme pays over 2 million claims per year for cataract surgery. These are quick outpatient procedures. They do not involve blood loss or much postoperative pain, but they are not minor procedures. Ophthalmic surgery can be a major life event. Establishing a professional relationship reduces anxiety and helps the patient prepare for surgery.

Psychological preparation

Giving information to the patient is just as important as getting information from the patient. An informed patient will be more calm, comfortable, and cooperative. The patient needs to know what to expect.

Informed consent

Informed consent is required. The anaesthetist should discuss the planned anaesthetic procedure, the risks, and any alternatives. This need not take more than a few minutes, but it should not be rushed. The discussion of risk should be guided by the medical history and physiologic status.

Risk assessment

Two important factors influencing outcome are the degree of illness of the patient and the degree of stress of the surgery. Patients with severe medical problems have higher risk and require more intensive evaluation before surgery. Patients having more invasive procedures also need more intensive studies. Preoperative evaluation of the ophthalmic patient is controversial because it usually involves the preparation of a high-risk patient for low-risk surgery.

Eye surgery patients are high-risk as a group. They tend to be old. Most have other risk factors such as diabetes, hypertension, and atherosclerosis. Cataract has been shown to be a marker for increased mortality. Ophthalmic surgery, however, is low-risk. Mortality after eye procedures is much lower than for the general surgical population. Eye surgery in patients with previous myocardial infarction does not pose the risk of myocardial re-infarction seen with general surgical procedures. Patients' chronic diseases have less effect on outcome with these procedures. Age and American Society of Anesthesiologists (ASA) class have not been shown to be significant risk factors for poor outcomes or unanticipated hospital admissions after outpatient ophthalmic surgery.

Planning perioperative management

There is controversy regarding the best preoperative management. Some say that because cataract extraction is a low-stress, no-blood-loss procedure, no preoperative evaluation is needed. Publication of a large, multicentre trial showed no effect of preoperative blood tests and electrocardiogram on postoperative outcome. Another opinion is that every patient must receive a full evaluation to include every possible test, to detect every possible finding, to institute every possible therapy, and to delay as long as possible, so that the patient can be in the best possible condition and have the lowest possible risk. Appropriate preoperative medical consultation is important. Malpractice litigation in cataract surgery finds negligence in medical consultation at about the same rate as negligence attributed to either local or general anaesthesia.

It is important not to ignore the risks. Neither do we want to reduce every risk to the lowest conceivable minimum. Our goal is to prepare the patient to present an acceptable lowest risk at surgery. Acceptable risk is determined by the medical care team with the informed consent of the patient. If a patient's condition would indicate inpatient admission for medical treatment, or if a reversible condition would likely lead to a perioperative complication, then the risk is not acceptable.

Guidelines for preoperative care

The goal is to develop guidelines that would encourage consistency of care and minimize disruption to patients and the operating room. The following guidelines are presented after review of literature and published guidelines.

Patient history

Previous hospitalizations and surgical procedures are reviewed. Allergies and drug sensitivities are noted. Latex allergy should be addressed specifically. A current list of medications is obtained. Of particular concern to the ophthalmologist is the patient with prostatic hypertrophy taking α-1 blockers such as tamsulosin. These patients are known to be at risk for intraoperative floppy iris syndrome with difficulty at the time of cataract surgery.

Patient factors that could impair the patient's ability to cooperate with surgery under local anaesthesia include:
- Dementia
- Deafness
- Language difficulty
- Restless leg syndrome
- Obstructive sleep apnoea
- Tremors
- Dizziness
- Claustrophobia

A preoperative patient questionnaire can be very helpful. A thorough review of the patient history will help perioperative planning and establishing a doctor–patient relationship.

Physical examination

Check for signs of major cardiac or pulmonary decompensation. Particular attention should be paid to positioning issues such as severe scoliosis or orthopnoea.

Laboratory studies

No routine screening tests have been shown to improve outcome. Laboratory studies should be determined on the basis of the results of the history and physical examination. As a general rule, the tests that a patient needs prior to ophthalmic procedures are the same as that which the patient would require at a routine exam if surgery were not planned. Tests are chosen when the results are likely to change management. Urgent medical management is obtained for results reaching critical limits.

Electrocardiogram (ECG)

- New chest pain, decreased exercise tolerance, clinical examination, palpitations, near-syncope, fatigue, or dyspnoea
- Tachycardia, bradycardia, or irregular pulse on
  - **Critical results**: signs of acute ischemia or injury, malignant arrhythmia, complete heart block, atrial fibrillation which is new, or with heart rate greater than 100bpm

Serum electrolytes
- History of severe vomiting or diarrhoea, poor oral intake, changes in diuretic management, arrhythmia
  - **Critical results**: sodium less than 120mmol/L or greater than 158mmol/L. Potassium less than 2.8mmol/L or greater than 6.2mmol/L

Urea nitrogen
- Signs or symptoms of renal de-compensation
  - **Critical result**: greater than 20mmole/L

Serum glucose
- Polydipsia, polyuria, and weight loss
  - **Critical results**: less than 46mg/dL or greater than 484mg/dL
- Haematocrit/haemoglobin
- History of bleeding, poor oral intake, fatigue, decreased exercise tolerance, tachycardia
  - **Critical results**: haematocrit less than 18% or greater than 61%. Haemoglobin less than 6.6mg/dL or greater than 19.9mg/dL

Ophthalmic evaluation

Visual acuity

The visual acuity of both eyes should be noted. Patients with poor vision in the non-operative eye face much greater potential functional loss. These patients have a higher anxiety level. If the patient is to be patched overnight, the physician should anticipate the increased need for postoperative assistance for a temporarily blind patient.

Axial length

The axial length of the globe should be assessed. When ultrasound measurements are available, the axial length should be noted. If no ultrasound is available, a myopic patient should be assumed to have an increased axial length. If a posterior staphyloma is present, the risks of injection anaesthesia may be dramatically increased. Preoperative glaucoma history, increased intra-ocular pressure, and increased axial length are important risk factors for suprachoroidal haemorrhage. The risk may be reduced with tighter control of intraoperative heart rate and preoperative intra-ocular pressure. Preoperative softening with a compression device may also decrease risk.

Cardiovascular evaluation

The American Heart Association and American College of Cardiology published guidelines for perioperative cardiovascular evaluation for non-cardiac surgery. Ophthalmic procedures such as cataract extraction are specifically identified as low-risk procedures. For these procedures, evaluation is focused on patients with major clinical predictors of risk. These major predictors generally mandate intensive management that often results in delay or cancellation of surgery until the cardiac problem is clarified and appropriately treated.

Recent myocardial infarction

Recent myocardial infarction (MI) with evidence of important ischaemic risk:

- The American College of Cardiology defines recent MI as less than or equal to 30 days. This is a much shorter period than the 3–6 months that have often been used as a guideline
- Indications for coronary angioplasty or coronary revascularization procedures are the same as if the patient were not having an ophthalmic procedure

Unstable or severe angina

This includes Canadian Class III or IV:

- Class III is defined as marked limitations of ordinary physical activity. Angina occurs on walking one to two blocks on the level or climbing one flight of stairs
- Class IV is defined as the inability to carry on any physical activity without discomfort—angina symptoms may be present at rest

Decompensated congestive cardiac failure

These patients normally cannot lie flat for a procedure.

Significant arrhythmia

These include:

- High-grade atrioventricular block such as complete heart block
- Symptomatic ventricular arrhythmia, and supraventricular arrhythmias with uncontrolled ventricular rate
- A careful evaluation for drug toxicity or metabolic derangement should be done
- Indications for cardiac pacing and antiarrhythmic therapy are the same as in the non-operative setting

Severe valvular disease

Symptomatic stenotic lesions are associated with severe congestive heart failure and shock.

- These may require percutaneous valvotomy or valve replacement
- Symptomatic regurgitant lesions can usually be stabilized with medical therapy
- Because ophthalmic procedures are not associated with significant bacteraemia, antibiotic prophylaxis is not recommended

Hypertension

Hypertension is a common problem in ophthalmic patients. Severe hypertension may lead to perioperative complications.

Degrees of hypertension have been defined:

- Stage 3 of severe hypertension is defined as a systolic of 180mmHg or more, or a diastolic of 110mmHg or more
- It is suggested to reschedule elective procedures in patients with sustained stage 3 hypertension at least for two weeks of antihypertensive therapy

Respiratory system evaluation

Ophthalmic procedures generally require that the patient lie flat comfortably and quietly. If the patient cannot lie flat, or if there is intractable cough, a perioperative complication is more likely. Special posture can be adopted (see 📖 Procedures requiring non-standard positioning, p. 358). Preoperative risk-reduction strategies include:
• Cessation of cigarette smoking
• Treatment of airflow obstruction with bronchodilators or steroids
• Administration of antibiotics for respiratory infections
• Patients should be assessed for sleep apnoea
• Intravenous sedation is often contraindicated in these patients
• For some patients, treatment with a mild stimulant such as caffeine can be helpful in keeping them awake and cooperative during a procedure

Endocrine system evaluation

Diabetes mellitus is very common in the ophthalmic surgical population.
• It is best if these patients can be done early in the morning with as little disturbance as possible to their usual daily routine
• Severe hyperglycaemia and hypoglycaemia are to be avoided
• Fasting blood glucose should be checked preoperatively
• Insulin therapy should be used, if needed, to keep the blood glucose in the range of 8mmole/L
• The potential for autonomic neuropathy needs to be considered, especially when elevating the patient from the supine position
Patients on long-term steroid therapy generally do not require 'stress-dose' steroid treatment for ophthalmic surgery.
• The patient should be given their normal dose of steroid on the day of surgery
• The physician should be alert to the occasional patient who may require additional glucocorticoid perioperatively
• Unexpected hypotension, fatigue, and nausea may be signs of a patient who needs additional steroid

Anticoagulant therapy and ophthalmic surgery

Many patients for ophthalmic surgery may be taking anticoagulant medications. Perioperative management of anticoagulant medications involves weighing the relative risks of thrombotic vs. haemorrhagic complications. Either of these results can be devastating to the patient.

- The risk of thrombotic complications depends on:
  - The indication for anticoagulation. Serious complications from arterial thromboembolic disease such as atrial fibrillation or valvular heart disease are much more common than complications from venous disease, such as deep venous thrombosis
  - The risk factors for thromboembolism in the individual, especially if and when the patient had a previous episode of thromboembolism
- The risk of haemorrhagic complications depends on:
  - The degree of anticoagulation
  - The haemorrhagic potential of the surgical procedure. Serious haemorrhagic complications are most probable in orbital and oculoplastic surgery, intermediate in vitreoretinal glaucoma, and corneal transplant and least likely in cataract surgery

A consensus is developing that cataract surgery may be safely performed while maintaining patients on anticoagulants. For intermediate risk procedures, the risk of surgical bleeding versus thrombotic complications must be weighed to determine if warfarin should be continued or stopped prior to surgery.

For high-risk cases for haemorrhage or thrombosis, cessation of warfarin or conversion to heparinization may be required. In those patients at higher risk for weaning from anticoagulants, the surgeon, internist/cardiologist, and patient should agree on a course of action.

Vision-threatening complications from needle-based blocks are exceedingly rare. Sub-Tenon's block or topical anaesthesia may be considered if feasible.

Conclusion

Appropriate preoperative preparation is an ethical requirement for the medical care team. A thorough preoperative evaluation will better prepare the patient for surgery, prevent cancellations and delays, and lead to better outcomes for our patients.

Further reading

Backer CL, Tinker JH, Robertson DM, Vlietstra RE. Myocardial reinfarction following local anesthesia for ophthalmic surgery. *Anesth. Analg.* 1980; 59(4): 257–62.

Flach AJ. Intraoperative floppy iris syndrome: pathophysiology, prevention, and treatment. *Trans. Am. Ophthalmol. Soc.* 2009; 107: 234–9.

Katz J, Feldman MA, Bass EB, Lubomski LH, Tielsch JM, Petty BG, Fleisher LA, Schein OD. Risks and benefits of anticoagulant and antiplatelet medication use before cataract surgery. Study of Medical Testing for Cataract Surgery Team. *Ophthalmology.* 2003; 110(9): 1784–8.

Langston RH. What is the risk of complications from cataract surgery in patients taking anticoagulants? *Cleve Clin. J. Med.* 2001 Feb; 68(2): 97–8.

Palda V. PRE-OPportunity knocks: a different way to think about the preoperative evaluation. *Am. Fam. Physician.* 2000 Jul 15; 62(2): 308–11.

Schein OD, Katz J, Bass EB, Tielsch JM, Lubomski LH, Feldman MA, Petty BG, Steinberg EP. The value of routine preoperative medical testing before cataract surgery. Study of Medical Testing for Cataract Surgery. *N. Engl. J. Med.* 2000 Jan 20; 342(3): 168–75.

Chapter 6

Needle-based orbital regional anaesthesia for adult ophthalmic surgery

Professor Steven Gayer

Introduction

Anaesthesia techniques for ophthalmological procedures can be subdivided into two categories:
- Those that render the globe akinetic (no muscle movements) via block of extra-ocular muscle (EOM) function.
- Those that do not affect globe motility (kinetic).

Selection of local anaesthesia

The selection of anaesthetic technique should be individualized based on:
- Specific patient needs
- The nature and extent of the procedure
- Both the anaesthetist's and surgeon's preferences and skills

Akinetic ophthalmic local anaesthesia techniques:
- Needle injection
- Sub-Tenon's injection

Kinetic ophthalmic local anaesthesia techniques:
- Topical anaesthesia
- Intra-cameral injection with or without sedation

Operations that can be accomplished via needle-based blocks

Aside from invasive oculo-plastic procedures that involve orbital bone and the need for general anaesthesia with paediatric cases, most eye surgery can be accomplished with needle-based anaesthesia. The following list is by no means comprehensive:
- Anterior segment surgery
  - Cataract (phacoemulsification, extracapsular, intracapsular)
  - Penetrating, lamellar, and endothelial keratoplasty (corneal transplantation)
  - Pterygium excision
- Glaucoma
  - Trabeculectomy
  - Trabeculotomy
  - Trabectome
- Retina
  - Scleral buckle
  - Vitrectomy
  - Epiretinal membrane peel
- Strabismus
- Facial plastics
- Evisceration
- Enucleation
- Orbital tumours
- Selected trauma cases

  Eye surgery conducted under general anaesthesia is often supplemented with a block prior to emergence to minimize postoperative discomfort. Anaesthetic blockade also:
- Suppresses the incidence of the oculocardiac reflex
- Provides postoperative pain management

- Many ophthalmologists opt for the operating milieu conferred by needle based anaesthesia—an immobile, fully anaesthetized eye—even for some procedures that can be accomplished with a kinetic technique.

Terminology

Akinetic ophthalmic anaesthesia is achieved with needle injection of local anaesthetic (LA) into the orbit. The terminology used to describe eye blocks may be somewhat confusing.

Traditional appellations

- Retrobulbar block:
  - This term, originating almost 100 years ago, was designed to indicate the ultimate position of the tip of the needle.
  - 'Retro' and 'bulbar' = behind the globe.
- Peribulbar block:
  - A newer form of needle block
  - First described in the 1980s
  - 'Peri' and 'bulbar' = around the globe
- Epibulbar, episcleral, peri-ocular, or parabulbar block:
  - Variant labels
  - In practice, many physicians by default refer any ophthalmic block as retrobulbar.

Newer appellations

More recent terminology may be less ambiguous. Instead of describing the relative position of the needle tip to the globe, it utilizes the muscle cone as the basis for nomenclature.

- Intraconal block:
  - Analogous to retrobulbar block
  - Injection of a small volume of LA inside of the muscle cone produces rapid onset of akinesia and analgesia
- Extraconal block:
  - Akin to peribulbar block
  - Injection of a larger volume of LA into the orbit, peripheral to the muscle cone.

Intraconal versus extraconal blocks

Most of the EOMs originate at the orbital apex in the Annulus of Zinn, extend anteriorly to their insertion points on the globe, and form a compartment within the orbit that resembles a cone.

- Intraconal (retrobulbar) block is accomplished by guiding a steeply angled apically directed needle from an insertion site near the inferotemporal margin of the orbital rim into the muscle cone (see Figure 6.1).

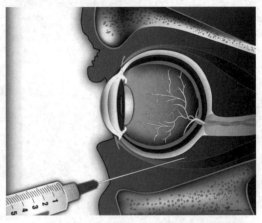

Fig. 6.1 Intraconal Block: Traditionally, a steeply angled, deeply placed injection has been referred to as a retrobulbar block. (Illustration by Jennifer Thomson, Bascom Palmer Eye Institute, University of Miami Miller School of Medicine).

- As delineated in the anatomy chapter, the muscle cone does not have a discrete septum that isolates the intraconal compartment from the extraconal space, so LA injected outside of the cone diffuses inward (and vice versa). An extraconal/peribulbar block is performed by directing a minimally angled needle fairly parallel to the globe to a shallow depth such that the tip remains outside of the cone (see Figure 6.2).

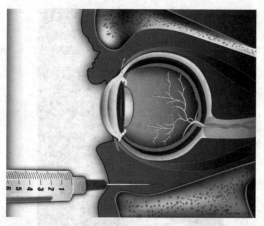

Fig. 6.2 Extraconal Block: LA injected peripheral to the EOM cone will diffuse inward and establish anesthesia. Also known as a peribulbar block. (Illustration by Jennifer Thomson, Bascom Palmer Eye Institute, University of Miami Miller School of Medicine).

- LA is deposited further from the key nerves with extraconal injection, thus requires more time and larger volumes for diffusion and has a longer latency of onset.
- Two key distinctions between intraconal and extraconal blocks are depth and angulation of needle placement. Theoretically, there is more potential for needle misadventure with intraconal versus extraconal anaesthesia since the tip may be directed toward and deep to the orbit's apex, an area densely packed with optic nerve, cranial nerves, major orbital vessels, and muscles. In contrast, extraconal block needles are guided towards the greater wing of the sphenoid bone, an area containing relatively few critical structures. Both are suitable means to achieve orbital anaesthesia (see Figure 6.3).

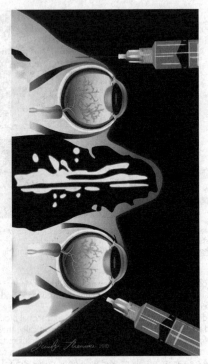

Fig. 6.3 Coronal view highlighting differences in depth and angulation of intraconal (lower image) and extraconal (upper image) blocks. Note that the intraconal needle travels underneath the globe, but appears to pass through it in this two-dimensional coronal view. (Illustration by Jennifer Thomson, Bascom Palmer Eye Institute, University of Miami Miller School of Medicine).

Intraconal block (see Figure 6.4)
- Steeply angled and deeply placed
- Directed in alignment with the bony orbital axis
- Needle tip aimed towards the orbital apex
- Lower volume of anaesthetic agent (1–3ml)
- Brisk advent of akinesia and analgesia
- Sparing of orbicularis oculi muscle
- May require separate facial nerve block for lid akinesia to prevent blepharospasm (lid squeezing)
- Greater potential for complications:
  - Globe perforation—posterior or inferior pole of the eye
  - Optic nerve sheath injection—brainstem anaesthesia, trauma
  - Intravascular injection—convulsions, apnoea, loss of consciousness

- • Retrobulbar haemorrhage
- • Postoperative diplopia
- Not recommended without training and experience
- Globe penetration or perforation may lead to permanent visual loss
- Brainstem anaesthesia may cause apnoea, dysrhythmia, cardiac arrest etc.

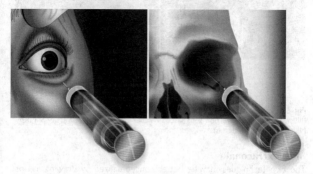

Fig. 6.4 Intraconal or retrobulbar block. Needle angle follows axis of the bony orbit. (Illustration by Jennifer Thomson, Bascom Palmer Eye Institute, University of Miami Miller School of Medicine).

Modified intraconal block

- Technique adapted to improve safety profile
- Shorter needle placed at lesser depth
- Needle inserted more laterally, further from globe and inferior EOMs
- No steep redirection of needle once it has passed the equator
- Needle angle is less acute, not aimed directly toward the orbital apex

Extraconal block (see Figure 6.5)

- Minimally angled, nearly parallel to globe
- Shallow needle depth
- Directed parallel to the optical axis
- Needle tip aimed towards the greater wing of the sphenoid bone
- Higher volume local anaesthetic agent (4–10cc)
- More gradual onset of akinesia and analgesia
- Orbicularis oculi function attenuated
- Dispersion of LA in the extraconal space:
  - • Blocks lid function
  - • Prevents blepharospasm (reflex lid squeezing)
  - • Therefore separate facial nerve block not required
- Lesser potential for significant complications
- Adverse consequences are nonetheless feasible
- Retrobulbar haemorrhage and globe penetration less likely if use single infero-lateral injection technique, avoiding superior aspect of orbit
- May be supplemented with a medial canthus block

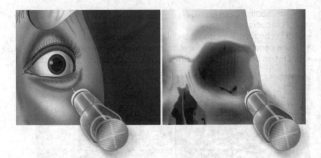

Fig. 6.5 Extraconal or peribulbar block. Needle angle parallels the globe.
(Illustration by Jennifer Thomson, Bascom Palmer Eye Institute, University of Miami Miller School of Medicine).

Intra/extraconal

The two techniques may be better conceptualized by drawing a loose analogy with subarachnoid and epidural anaesthesia (see Table 6.1)

- There are noted similarities in terms of:
  - Depth of injection
  - Volume
  - Speed
  - Density of block

Table 6.1 Ophthalmic blocks analogy with neuraxial block

	Intraconal/subarachnoid	Extraconal/epidural
Needle depth	Deep	More shallow
Cone/dura	Through	Peripheral to
LA volume	Lower	Higher
Latency of onset	Quick	More gradual
Density of initial block	Dense	Less so

Needle considerations

There are an abundant variety of needles available for use. Their properties differ based upon shape, length, bevel, and gauge.

Shape

- Straight:
  - Generally inexpensive and readily available
- Curved:
  - Intended to align with the contour of the globe
  - Spectrum of globe sizes and shapes renders uncertainty as to final position of needle tip
  - Largely abandoned, not commonly used now

Length

- Traditionally 38mm (1.5ins)
- The apex of the orbit contains little adipose tissue. It is densely packed with optic nerve and muscle origins
- Potential to reach apex of the orbit with a deeply seated 38mm needle is higher, enhancing prospect of:
  - Optic nerve trauma
  - Sheath injection
  - Brainstem anaesthesia
  - Muscle trauma
  - More
- 25mm (1in) to 32mm (1.25in) needles
- Greatly reduced likelihood of the needle encroaching into the orbital apex
- The pyramidal-shaped bony orbit narrows as it extends posteriorly towards its apex. The lateral rectus muscle comes to lie directly adjacent to the orbital bone, ablating the extraconal space. An intended extraconal block with a 25–32mm needle (placed without angulation towards the orbital apex), may, in fact, result in an unintended intraconal injection.
- Needles <25mm (1in)
- Anterior periocular block
- Commonly 5/8inch (15mm)
- Require higher volume (8–10cc)
- Directed toward the orbital floor
- Diminished potential for injection into the deep orbit
- Generally associated with longer latency of block onset
- Supplemental injection may be required to achieve complete akinesia

Bevel and gauge

Upon insertion, the bevel of the needle should face the globe, increasing the distance of the tip from the sclera.

- Sharp bevelled, narrow gauge (27–30g)
  - Easier to insert
  - Less pain upon entry
  - Penetrate tissue more readily
  - Scleral penetration may go unnoticed

- Blunt bevel, wider gauge (23–25g)
  - May have better tactile feedback or 'feel'
  - More discomfort upon insertion
  - May increase indication for pre-injection sedation/analgesic
  - Compared with finer, sharper needles, blunt larger gauge needles may require more force in order to unintentionally penetrate sclera, decreasing likelihood of needle penetration (remains controversial)
- In theory, observation of globe movement during placement of the needle may be indicative of impending scleral perforation, signalling need to withdraw and reassess (alternatively, movement may be due to engagement of inferior rectus or inferior oblique muscles)
- Injury incurred from inadvertent penetration of the globe by a blunt-bevel, lower-gauge needle may be more extensive than that from a narrower, sharper needle
- Regardless of bevel or gauge, careful observation of the globe during slow, deliberate insertion of the needle is warranted. Needle excursion should be halted upon any indication of globe movement

Needle entry sites

Needle blocks have been performed at nearly every conceivable position around the eye. Access is usually achieved transcutaneously or by transconjunctival injection.

Traditional entry site

- The landmark for the traditional insertion site for both intraconal and extraconal blocks is pinpointed by dropping a plumb line from the lateral margin of the pupil's limbus down to the area just superior to the inferior orbital rim.
- This location is often referred to as the 'one-third:two-thirds' point as it is situated by the inferior orbital rim approximately two-thirds of the way from the medial canthus (see Figure 6.6 point A).

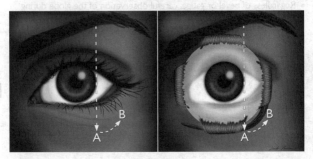

Fig. 6.6 Inferotemporal needle insertion site. Point A: Traditional location derived by dropping a plumb line from the lateral limbal margin of a globe in neutral gaze. Point B: Modified entry site shifted towards the inferotemporal corner. (Illustration by Jennifer Thomson, Bascom Palmer Eye Institute, University of Miami Miller School of Medicine).

Modified traditional insertion site

- The inferior rectus muscle as well as the inferior oblique muscle and its neurovascular bundle may be encountered by a needle introduced at the traditional entry point
- Inadvertent injection of LA into these thin muscles can induce local scarring and result in a restrictive postoperative strabismus. This may resolve spontaneously over a period of days to months, but may also be permanent, requiring surgical correction
  - Use of lower concentration local anaesthetics and hyaluronidase additive may lessen the likelihood of postoperative diplopia
- Injection into either of the two muscles can be avoided by shifting the needle insertion site more laterally along the inferotemporal margin toward the corner of the orbit (see Figure 6.6 point B)

Superior injection sites

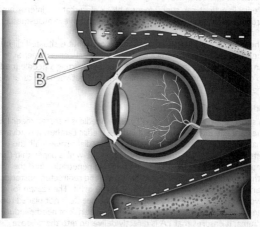

Fig. 6.7 Superior approach: Due to limited space and prominence of orbital rim, a parallel approach (A) is not advisable. The needle should be angled upwards (B). (Illustration by Jennifer Thomson, Bascom Palmer Eye Institute, University of Miami Miller School of Medicine).

- The roof of the bony orbit is much less angled than its floor, lying more parallel to the coronal plane; therefore a needle placed into the superior orbit can penetrate deeper and further than the same length needle introduced into the inferior orbit (see Figure 6.7)
- The globe is not centred in the orbit, but is situated higher, more proximate to the orbital roof. Therefore, the ingress space for a needle introduced into the superior orbit is more constricted than that available at the inferior orbital rim (see Figure 6.7)
- The superior orbital rim is more protuberant due to expansion of the frontal sinus above it. Because of this and the diminished space in the superior orbit, initially needles should be placed with an upward angulation (see Figure 6.7)
- The superior oblique muscle, its tendon, and its delicate trochlear apparatus can be encountered and injured by a needle introduced into the superonasal orbit. The ophthalmic artery, the superior ophthalmic vein, and branches of the nasociliary nerve are also present in this region
- The superior orbit contains a greater preponderance of branches of the ophthalmic artery and vein. Increased vascularity contributes to an enhanced risk of needle-induced bleeding
- Early descriptions of techniques for peribulbar blocks called for a combination of inferior and superior injections. This has been largely abandoned due to:
  - The considerations described above
  - Given sufficient time, a single, higher volume, inferiorly placed injection provides excellent anaesthesia

Medial insertion sites

- Medial injections can supplement a block placed at the infero-temporal orbital rim or be used as a primary means to achieve anaesthesia of the eye.
- The globe is not directly centred in the orbit, but is situated slightly to the temporal side, creating a fat-filled paranasal compartment.
- An extraconal injection can be achieved by inserting a needle medial to the caruncle or along the semilunaris fold between the caruncle and the globe.

Medial canthal technique

- A short, sharp (0.5–1.0in, 25–30 gauge) needle is inserted medial to the caruncle into the tunnel behind the medial canthus. It is advanced shallowly until contact is made with the medial orbital wall, then retracted slightly (1–2mm). At this point, the wall is paper-thin (lamina papyracea) so care must be taken to avoid penetrating into the ethmoid sinus. The needle is then angled and redirected posteriorly, parallel to the medial wall and floor of the orbit. The reason for this two-step manoeuvre is to assure that the needle is not placed too medially, putting the medial rectus muscle at risk of needle-induced trauma. It ensures that LA is directly delivered into the adipose compartment adjacent to the medial rectus muscle.

Medial canthus episcleral block (needle sub-Tenon's technique)

- Sharp, medial/nasal-directed needle placed into the semilunaris fold between the caruncle and the globe.
- The globe often rotates considerably medially during insertion. The needle is then lifted into a position facing directly posterior until a click-sensation is discerned. This occurs as the needle engages and then passes through the medial check ligament into either the extraconal space medial to the medial rectus muscle or inside Tenon's capsule, depending on length of needle used. Upon reaching this point, the globe rotates back into neutral gaze position and local anaesthetic is then injected.

Globe considerations

There are a number of variables related to the globe itself that are important to take into consideration prior to embarking upon a needle-based eye block. These include the size, shape, and position of the globe (see Figure 6.8).

- An atypically long or misshapen or deeply recessed eye may have enhanced risk for inadvertent penetration by the needle

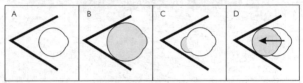

Fig. 6.8 Globe considerations: A: Normal. B,C,D: Risk of penetration is enhanced by a larger eye(B), staphyloma (C), Marked globe recession (D). (Illustration by Rick Stratton, Bascom Palmer Eye Institute, University of Miami Miller School of Medicine).

Size

- The typical globe's anterior–posterior dimension (axial length) is approximately 22–24mm
- Biometry of globe length is commonly obtained via ultrasound of the eye (A-scan)
- This assesses the distance from the corneal surface to the anterior aspect of the retina
- Axial length—tends to be longer in the presence of:
  - Myopia (spherical equivalents of –3.00 or greater)
  - Staphyloma
  - An *in-situ* scleral buckle
- An elongated globe may be at higher risk for penetration at the inferior pole or the eye's posterior aspect by a steeply angled, deep intraconal injection (see Figure 6.8B)
- A shallow, minimally angled extraconal block is less likely to reach the posterior surface of the globe, but may pierce the globe's inferior pole
- It is useful to obtain the axial length, when available, prior to performing a needle-based block

Shape

- A staphyloma is an abnormal outpouching of the globe
- Although they can occur anywhere on the globe, they are typically found at the posterior aspect by the insertion of the optic nerve. They may be noted on an ultrasound report
- The presence of a staphyloma increases the risk of needle penetration (see Figure 6.8C)

Position

- Globe orbit relationship is an important consideration
- The globe's position within the orbit can be assessed by noting the eye's surface anatomy

- An enophthalmic (recessed) globe is at increased risk of needle penetration
- The combination of marked enophthalmos and increased axial length is particularly concerning and should be noted on physical examination
- A large, deeply recessed globe in a small orbit is at increased risk of needle injury (see Figure 6.8D)

Gaze position

- Traditionally, patients were instructed to gaze upward and nasally inward
- This has been abandoned in favour of keeping the eye in neutral gaze position
- Upward and inward focus stretches the optic nerve tautly and places it in the path of a needle placed in retrobulbar fashion
- The nerve may be traumatized by the needle or local anaesthetic agent may be injected along the optic nerve sheath (orbital epidural)
- This position also places the macula in the needle's trajectory
- Neutral gaze keeps the optic nerve lax and behind the globe
- The optic nerve passes through the optic canal then exits the skull through the optic foramen situated in the supero-medial wall of the orbit. From here it travels forward to enter the posterior aspect of the globe
- Within the orbit the globe sits slightly more to the lateral side
- Therefore, in theory, with the globe in neutral gaze position the optic nerve can be completely avoided by infero-temporal placement of a needle in such a way that the tip does not cross the plane formed by an imaginary plumb line dropped through the pupil (see Figure 6.9)

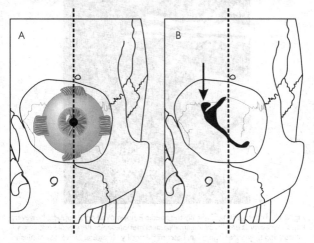

Fig. 6.9 Potential of reaching the optic nerve is minimized by keeping the needle tip lateral to this imaginary plane. (Arrow indicates optic canal). (Illustration by Rick Stratton, Bascom Palmer Eye Institute, University of Miami Miller School of Medicine).

Tether testing

- A controversial manoeuvre. This performed in order to reassure that the needle has not engaged the sclera and penetrated or perforated the globe. Those who practice this manoeuvre instruct the patient to briefly gaze laterally once the needle is *in situ*, just prior to injection of LA
  - Medial movement of the globe is discouraged as it may bring the optic nerve closer to the needle tip
- Alternatively, others advocate gentle parallel non-torqued movement of the needle to provide confidence that it is not tethered in the globe (see Figure 6.10)
- Finally, many ophthalmic anaesthetists believe that once the needle is in position it is not acceptable to move at all

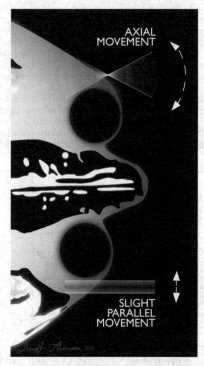

Fig. 6.10 Tether-testing: Typically the needle is not moved once in place; however, if this maneuver is employed, minimal parallel motion diminishes needle excursion. (Illustration by Jennifer Thomson, Bascom Palmer Eye Institute, University of Miami Miller School of Medicine).

Oculocompression

Short needle extraconal blocks are prone to retrograde flow of LA into the lower lid cul-de-sac behind the orbital septum. Local anaesthetic mass effect with intraconal blocks may place pressure on the posterior globe. In either case, dispersion of LA and softening of the eye can be augmented by several means:

- Applying digital pressure on the lower lid while injecting.
  - Alternatively, one can have an assistant place two fingers gently on the medial aspect of the lower lid while injecting. Take care to provide intermittent, gentle pressure as continuous pressure may compromise vascular perfusion.
- Digital message after completion of the block.
- Use of an ocular compression device after block.
  - Tungsten or mercury bag designed for this purpose (Mercury is no longer permissible in many healthcare facilities.)
  - Honan balloon.

Facial nerve block

The forward diffusion of the greater volume of local anaesthetics used with an extraconal block provides a degree of eyelid akinesia and attenuation of the ability to squeeze the lids.

- In contrast, a lower volume intraconal block does not suppress lid function. In addition to the primary anaesthetic injection, a second block of the facial nerve branches that supply the orbicularis oculi may be indicated
- The 7th (VIIth) cranial nerve can be blocked at any point along its excursion from the stylomastoid foramen to the orbicularis oculi
  - Distal injection of LA in the area where the facial nerve exits the stylomastoid foramen (Nadbath block) can lead to transient hemifacial paresis which may be misinterpreted as a stroke. Due to the proximity of the glossopharyngeal and vagus nerves, dysphagia, drooling, hoarseness, and more can occur (enthusiasm for this technique has waned)
  - A traditional Van Lint block was accomplished by injecting LA close to the orbital rim along the upper and lower lids. This can be painful and cause bleeding into the eyelids, so has been largely abandoned in favour of a modified technique
  - A proximal injection of a peau d'orange of LA by a needle approximately 1cm from the most temporal part of the lateral orbital rim, directed perpendicular to the skull just above periosteum, is a preferred method (modified Van Lint block). Digital pressure is then applied to spread the LA subcutaneously
- Facial nerve block to reduce the incidence of blepharospasm (tight eyelid squeezing) should be considered for:
  - Corneal transplantation surgery
  - Repair of traumatic eye injuries via regional anaesthesia
  - For those patients that cannot tolerate a lid speculum

Conclusion

Needle-based blocks are a highly effective and safe means to achieve optimal operating conditions for patients and surgeons. Thorough knowledge of orbital anatomy and geometric aspects of needle placement coupled with experience are requisite. Recent studies have explored the potential for ultrasound-guided needle-based ophthalmic regional anaesthesia. This technology may be useful for teaching safe techniques and may have a role in the future.

Further reading

Fanning G. Orbital regional anesthesia. *Ophthalmology Clinics of North America*. 2006; 19(2): 221–32.

Gayer S. Ophthalmic Anesthesia. *American Society of Anesthesiologists Refresher Courses In Anesthesiology*. 2006; 34(5): 55–63.

Gayer S. Ophthalmic Anesthesia: More Than Meets the Eye. In: Gallagher C, Martinez-Ruix R, and Lubarsky D eds. *Anesthesia Unplugged. A Step-by-Step Guide to Techniques and Procedures*. 2007; McGraw Hill Medical, 345–65.

Kumar CM. Needle-based blocks for 21st-century ophthalmology. *Acta. Ophthalmol.* 2010; Epub ahead of print.

Chapter 7

Cannula-based sub-Tenon's block for adult ophthalmic surgery

Professor Chandra M. Kumar

Introduction

The sub-Tenon's block was first described in the 19th century and was later reintroduced into clinical practice in the early 1990s as a simple, effective, and safe alternative to needle blocks. The technique involves the introduction of a blunt cannula under the Tenon's capsule and the injection of a local anaesthetic agent of choice to achieve anaesthesia and akinesia.

The use of sub-Tenon's block in some countries, especially the UK, is very high and preferred by ophthalmologists as well as anaesthetists over needle blocks. In contrast, needle blocks are favoured in the US. The technique may be used for a wide variety of ophthalmic surgical procedures.

The limitations and complications of sub-Tenon's anaesthesia have become better known in recent years.

The purpose of this chapter is to describe the basic knowledge required to perform the sub-Tenon's block, its limitations, and complications.

Anatomy

Before contemplating to perform any orbital block; one must have a comprehensive understanding of the basic sciences and techniques behind regional orbital blocks. The knowledge of globe anatomy, Tenon's capsule and its surrounding structures must also be mastered (see 📖 Tenon's capsule, p. 30).

Globe movements are controlled by four rectus muscles (inferior, lateral, medial, and superior) and two oblique muscles (superior and inferior). These muscles arise from the Annulus of Zinn at the apex of the orbit and they insert anterior to the equator of the globe and form an incomplete muscle cone. Almost all nerves and vessels supplying the globe and its surrounding structures enter the cone. The branches of the superior division of the oculomotor nerve (IIIrd nerve) supply the superior rectus and the levator palpebrae muscle. Branches of the inferior division of the oculomotor nerve supply the medial rectus, the inferior rectus and the inferior oblique muscles. The abducens nerve (VIth nerve) supplies the lateral rectus. The trochlear nerve (IVth nerve) lies outside and above the annulus and then enters the cone to supply the superior oblique muscle. Conjunctival sensations are mediated mainly through the nasociliary nerve (corneal, perilimbal, and the superonasal quadrant of the peripheral conjunctiva). The remainder of the peripheral conjunctiva is dissipated through the lacrimal, frontal, and infra-orbital nerves coursing outside the muscle cone.

The fascial sheath (Tenon's capsule) is a dense fibrous layer of elastic connective tissue surrounding the globe and extra-ocular muscles in the anterior orbit (Figure 7.1). It originates at the Annulus of Zinn and extends anteriorly blending with the connective tissue sheaths of the undersurface of all rectus and oblique muscles. It thus forms a socket for the eyeball. The Tenon's capsule is very tough in children and adults but becomes very thin in the elderly. There are numerous delicate bands of connective tissue in the sub-Tenon's space and these can resist the smooth insertion of a sub-Tenon cannula. The penetration of Tenon's capsule by the rectus muscles arbitrarily divides the capsule into anterior and posterior portions. The Tenon's capsule is adherent to the sclera in the anterior part for about 1.5–3mm from the limbus. The conjunctiva is also fused with the Tenon's capsule in this part. Therefore, the dissection to enter the Tenon's space is made 5–10mm away from the limbus. The posterior part of the Tenon's capsule passes around to the optic nerve, separating the globe from the contents of the retrobulbar space. The sheath fuses with the dura surrounding the optic nerve and with the sclera where the nerve enters the globe. Tenon's capsule is pierced by the ciliary nerves and vessels and by the vortex veins.

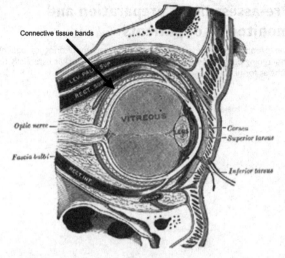

Fig. 7.1 Sub-Tenon's space showing multiple connective tissue bands. Reproduced with permission from Gray, Henry. Anatomy of the Human Body. Philadelphia: Lea & Febiger, 1918; Bartleby.com, 2000. Figure 891. www.bartleby.com/107/. Accessed 17th January 2012.

Pre-assessment, preparation and monitoring of patients

The preoperative assessment, preparation and monitoring of patients undergoing ophthalmic surgery under sub-Tenon's block is essentially the same as for needle-based blocks.

A standard sub-Tenon's technique

A standard sub-Tenon's technique

Access to the sub-Tenon's space through the inferonasal quadrant is the most common approach because the placement of the cannula in this quadrant allows good fluid distribution superiorly while avoiding the area of surgery and reducing the risk of damage to the vortex veins.

- After instillation of topical LA drops (proxymetacaine 0.5% or tetracaine 1%), a specially formulated 5% aqueous povidone iodine solution is instilled
- An eyelid speculum or an assistant's finger is used to keep the eyelids apart
- The patient is asked to look upwards and outwards, to expose the inferonasal quadrant and the conjunctiva and the Tenon's capsule are gripped with a non-toothed forceps (Moorfields forceps) 5–10mm away from the limbus
- A small incision is made with blunt-tipped Westcott scissors to expose the sclera
- A posterior, metal, blunt and curved sub-Tenon cannula (Figure 7.2a) (19G, 25mm long) is inserted along the curvature of the globe and 3–5cc of local anaesthetic agent is injected slowly
- If a resistance is encountered, gentle pressure is applied with hydro-dissection, usually helps in advancing the cannula. The resistance felt during insertion of the cannula may be due to the presence of interconnective tissue bands. If the hydro-dissection does not help or the resistance encountered is too great, it is advisable to reposition or reintroduce the cannula

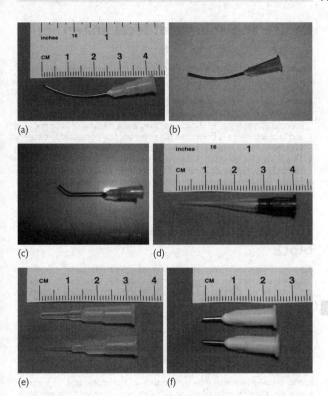

Fig. 7.2 a, metal, 2.54cm, curved, blunt, end hole (posterior sub-Tenon); b, flexible, 3cm long (Helica flexible); c, metal 2.3 cm long (triport metal); d, flexible 21G, 1.8cm long (mid sub-Tenon flexible cannula); e, flexible 1.2 cm long (Greenbaum's anterior plastic cannula); f, metal 0.6 cm long (ultrashort metal cannula).

There are also a variety of sub-Tenon's cannulae as illustrated in Figure 7.2.

There are no comparative data to support either the use of any particular sub-Tenon's cannula or site of access to any particular quadrant, but the superonasal route is thought to be potentially more hazardous because of the vascular, neuronal and muscular contents in that area.

There are other variations of the sub-Tenon's technique that relate to the site of access to the sub-Tenon's space including inferolateral, superotemporal, or medial episcleral.

Choice and volume of local anaesthetic agent

Anaesthesia and akinesia are determined by the properties of the LA agent, but more directly by the proximity to the sensory and motor nerves.

- 2% lidocaine is the most commonly used agent and is considered the gold standard. Other LA agents such as articaine, etidocaine, prilocaine, mepivacaine, levobupivacaine, and a mixture of lidocaine and bupivacaine have been used but there are few comparative data available on the relative effectiveness of various agents
- There is a wide variation in the use of volume of LA for sub-Tenon's block. The volumes vary from 1–11cc but most clinicians use 3–5cc
- Smaller volumes will usually provide globe anaesthesia but larger volumes are required if akinesia is desirable

The use of adjuvant during sub-Tenon's block

Adjuvant drugs are discussed elsewhere (see 📖 Additives, pp. 64–65).

Vasoconstrictors are commonly mixed with LA solution to increase the intensity and duration of block, and to minimize bleeding from small vessels.

- A short duration of anaesthesia is possible without addition of vasoconstrictor to lidocaine
- The use of epinephrine-containing solutions is usually avoided in elderly patients suffering from cerebrovascular and cardiovascular diseases.

Tachycardia induced by exogenous epinephrine may produce ischaemia

Hyaluronidase is an enzyme, which reversibly liquefies the interstitial barrier between cells by depolymerization of hyaluronic acid to a tetrasaccharide, thereby enhancing the diffusion of molecules through tissue planes.

- The amount of hyaluronidase mixed with the local anaesthetic varies from 0.5–150IU/cc.
- There is conflicting evidence that hyaluronidase improves the effectiveness and the quality of sub-Tenon's block. However, if hyaluronidase is used, it should not exceed 15IU/cc.

Advantages of sub-Tenon's block

The sub-Tenon's block not only reduces the well-known severe complications related to needle-based blocks but also provides reliable anaesthesia and has the potential for further supplementation for prolonged anaesthesia and postoperative pain relief. Numerous studies have demonstrated its relative effectiveness compared to retrobulbar, peribulbar, and topical anaesthesia. Sub-Tenon's block has been used for a large number of ophthalmic surgical procedures including:

- Cataract surgery
- Vitreoretinal surgery
- Panretinal photocoagulation
- Strabismus surgery
- Trabeculectomy
- Optic nerve sheath fenestration
- Chronic pain management and therapeutic delivery of drugs
- May be used safely in patients receiving anticoagulants and antiplatelet agents provided clotting results are in the normal therapeutic range

Limitations of sub-Tenon's block

Although the sub-Tenon's block is used for a wide variety of ophthalmic procedures, it does have limitations (see Table 7.1).

- The globe usually appears red and swollen due to subconjunctival haemorrhage and chemosis (see later) and they frequently occur during sub-Tenon's block
- Movements of the globe due to incomplete akinesia may cause problem during ophthalmic surgery (viscocanalostomy) which requires a still eye
- Some glaucoma surgeons dislike sub-Tenon's block although it has been used successfully for glaucoma surgery
- The block may be difficult to perform in patients who have had previous sub-Tenon's block in the same quadrant, previous retinal detachment and strabismus surgery, eye trauma, conjunctival disease (severe ocular pemphigoid), and infection to the orbit

Table 7.1 Limitations

Limitations
Previous sub-Tenon's block in the same quadrant
Previous extensive vitreoretinal surgery
Previous repeated strabismus surgery
Eye trauma
Infection to the orbit
Severe ocular pemphigoid
Surgery requiring complete akinesia (viscocanalostomy)
Surgery where chemosis and subconjunctival haemorrhage may compromise the outcome of surgery (glaucoma filtration surgery)

Minor complications

Pain during injection

The incidence of pain during sub-Tenon's injection with posterior metal cannulae is reported in up to 44% of patients. Preoperative explanation of the procedure, good surface anaesthesia, gentle technique, slow injection of warm LA agent, and reassurance are considered good practice and may reduce the discomfort and anxiety during the injection.

Chemosis

Chemosis signifies anterior injection of the anaesthetic agent and varies from 25–60%. This usually occurs if:
- A large volume of LA is injected
- Tenon's capsule is not dissected properly
- Shorter cannulae are used
- Chemosis may not be localized but usually resolves after the application of digital pressure

Subconjunctival haemorrhage

Fine vessels are inevitably and unintentionally severed during conjunctival dissection. The incidence (and severity) of subconjunctival haemorrhage varies from 20–100% and depends on the cannula used. This can be minimized by careful dissection avoiding damage to fine vessels. The use of cautery does not seem to help.

Leakage of local anaesthetic agent

Forward leakage of anaesthetic agent during injection is commonly observed. This occurs if the dissection of the sub-Tenon's capsule is not complete or if there is a resistance to injection. Careful dissection of Tenon's capsule should be performed. Tenting tissue over the dissection serves to increase resistance and decreases retrograde flow.

Akinesia and anaesthesia

Akinesia and anaesthesia is volume-dependent and if 4–5cc of LA agent is injected, most patients develop akinesia. However, superior oblique muscle and lid movements may remain active in a small but significant number of patients.

Sight- and life-threatening complications

Sight- and life-threatening complications have been reported. Most of these complications (see Table 7.2) have been reported as case reports and involved the use of long posterior metal sub-Tenon's cannula. The reported complications are:

- Short-lived muscle paresis
- Orbital and retrobulbar haemorrhage
- Scleral perforation
- Trauma to inferior and medial rectus muscles leading to restrictive functions resulting in diplopia
- Optic neuropathy
- Afferent pupillary and accommodation defects
- Retinal and choroidal vascular occlusion
- Cases of central spread of the LA agent leading to cardiorespiratory collapse. The mechanism of central spread is not clear, but perhaps spread of the injected LA agent into the subarachnoid space through the optic nerve sheath or back tracking of the LA agent through one of the orbital foramina are possible explanations
- Death associated with sub-Tenon's block

Table 7.2 Sight- and life-threatening complications of sub-Tenon's block

Complications	Possible mechanism	Risk factors	Incidence	Prevention	Treatment
Brainstem anaesthesia	Injection into the optic nerve sheath Unintentional perforation of Tenon's capsule and spread of LA to CNS through one of the orbital foramen	Deep posterior injection	Unknown	Adhere to basic anatomy, use shorter sub-Tenon's cannulae	Extensive cardiorespiratory support
Globe penetration	Improper dissection	Inexperienced user, poor technique, previous surgery	Unknown	Careful use of technique and adhere to basic anatomy	Immediate senior ophthalmic opinion
Intraorbital, orbital and/or retrobulbar haemorrhage	Trauma to blood vessel Rupture of sclerotic blood vessel	Patients receiving aspirin or clopidogrel Inappropriate technique	Unknown	Adhere to anatomy	Immediate oculocompression, ophthalmologic opinion and decompression surgery
Retinal ischaemia	Increase in IOP Retrobulbar haemorrhage Compression of blood vessel	High volume of LA Glaucoma Compromised circulation to retinal artery	Unknown	Void deep posterior injection	Ophthalmic opinion

(continued)

Table 7.2 (Contd.)

Complications	Possible mechanism	Risk factors	Incidence	Prevention	Treatment
Optic nerve damage	Direct trauma Optic neuropathy	Posterior injection High concentration of LA	Unknown	Avoid deep posterior injection, use recommended dose of appropriate LA	Ophthalmic opinion
Rectus muscle dysfunction	Direct trauma to muscle Injection of LA into the muscle Prolonged exposure of rectus muscle fibres with LA agent	Not known	Unknown	Proper placement of cannula Adhere to anatomy Avoid forceful injection	Ophthalmic opinion
Orbital swelling	Infection Excessive dose of hyaluronidase	Poor technique	Unknown	Aseptic technique, use recommended dose of hyaluronidase	Antibiotics, steroids and ophthalmic opinion

Intra-ocular pressure and pulsatile ocular blood flow

- The rise in intra-ocular pressure (IOP) after administration of sub-Tenon's block is small or even non-significant. However, there is a decrease in the pulsatile ocular blood flow during the sub-Tenon's anaesthesia (14%); therefore, caution is required in the management of patients whose ocular circulation may be compromised.

Conclusion

The sub-Tenon's block is a simple, effective, versatile and relatively safe technique but sight- and life-threatening complications can occur. This block has been used in most routine ophthalmic surgery but there a few limitations. A thorough knowledge of anatomy and understanding of the underlying principles is essential before embarking on this technique.

Further reading

Dutton JJ. *Atlas of clinical and surgical orbital anatomy.* Philadelphia: W.B. Saunders Co Ltd, 1994.

Kumar CM, Dodds C. Sub-Tenon's anesthesia. *Ophthalmol. Clin. North America.* 2006: 19; 209–19.

Kumar CM, Williamson S, Manickam B. A review of sub-Tenon's block: current practice and recent development. *Eur. J. Anaesthesiol.* 2005; 22: 567–77.

Kumar CM, Eid H, Dodds C. Sub-Tenon's anaesthesia: complications & their prevention. *Eye.* 2011: 25(6); 697–703.

Local anaesthesia for intraocular surgery. The Royal College of Anaesthetists and The Royal College of Ophthalmologists, 2001.

Snell RS, Lemp MA. *Clinical anatomy of the eye.* Boston: Blackwell Scientific Publications, 1989.

Stevens JD. A new local anesthesia technique for cataract extraction by one quadrant sub-Tenon's infiltration. *Br. J. Ophthalmol.* 1992; 76: 670–4.

Intra-ocular pressure and pulsatile ocular blood flow

Conclusion

Further reading

Ophthalmic topical anaesthesia

Dr Howard Palte

Introduction

The growing appeal of topical anaesthesia in cataract surgery is due in part to its distinct advantages of simplicity, minimal pain on administration, absence of significant systemic complications and a rapid postoperative recovery. Alternative techniques aim to circumvent the potential for topical-induced corneal epithelial toxicity.

Timeline

Koller first described the use of topical anaesthesia in 1884. Cocaine was associated with a marked stinging sensation upon instillation and caused corneal haziness, thus it was largely abandoned in favour of ether general anaesthesia. Over 100 years later, Fichman repopularized the topical anaesthesia technique with modern local anaesthetic agents.

- 5th century BC: early description cataract extraction—'couching'.
- 1884: Koller—topical cocaine—facilitated anterior chamber surgery
- 1884: Knapp—retrobulbar anaesthesia—akinesia. Blindness and toxic cocaine reactions.
- 1905: procaine—synthetic cocaine analogue
- 1943: lignocaine (lidocaine)—greater stability
- 1949: Atkinson—addition hyaluronidase
- 1965: bupivacaine—longer duration—cardiotoxic
- 1972: cataract phacoemulsification
- 1991: Fichman—topical anaesthesia for cataract surgery
- 1992: Stevens—sub-Tenon's block
- 1995: Gillis—intra-cameral anaesthesia

Mechanism of action

It is important to understand the sensory supply of the anterior part of the orbit before embarking on topical anaesthesia.

- Cornea—sensation derived from conjunctiva, episclera and sclera
  - Branches of ophthalmic division of trigeminal nerve (Vth nerve)
  - Long and short ciliary
  - Nasociliary
  - Lacrimal
- Terminal unmyelinated axons terminate in dense plexus of sub-Bowman's area
- Reversible blockade of sodium channels
- Prevent propagation action potentials in the cornea, conjunctiva, and sclera
- Nerve endings superficial—corneal epithelium permeable to lipid and aqueous soluble substances

Indications

Surgical
- Usually cataract extraction.
- Selective anterior vitrectomy with intra-cameral anaesthesia.
- Trabeculectomy with intra-cameral anaesthesia.

Surgeon
- Tolerant of eye movements (absence of akinesia)
- Cognisant of persistent light/tactile perception

Patient
- Cooperative
- Able to fix gaze
- Tolerant of sensations related to ocular manipulation
- Long axial length
- Active anticoagulation/bleeding diathesis

Relative contraindications

Surgical factors
- Extensive ocular manipulation (such as with 'white' or dense cataract).
- Floppy iris syndrome is common with those men who use 5α reductase agents for benign prostatic hypertrophy (BPH).
- Poor pupillary response to mydriatics and/or planned pupil-stretching or use of iris hooks.

Patient factors
- Anxiety
- Language barrier
- Hearing impairment
- Mental impairment
- Uncontrolled head tremor
- Children

Topical anaesthesia techniques

Modalities (see Table 8.1)

- Aqueous eye drops
- Viscous eye drops
- Eye drops + intra-cameral injection
- Eye drops + LA-soaked ophthalmic sponges placed in conjunctival fornix ('deep topical')
- Eye drops + LA-gel
- LA-soaked ophthalmic sponge to limbus/peri-limbal zone
- 'Bloomberg ring'
- LA-soaked circumferential corneal ring
- Cryo-anaesthesia:
  - Cold pack + irrigation with iced balanced salt solution

Efficacy

High

- Gel
- LA-soaked ophthalmic sponges
- Drops + gel
- Drops + intra-cameral injection

Intermediate

- Cryo-anaesthesia

Low

- Drops

Intra-cameral anaesthesia

- Used in conjunction with topical drops
- Paracentesis incision
- 0.5ml preservative-free 1% lignocaine
- Facilitates iris manipulation/anterior vitrectomy
- Endothelial injury (debatable)

Limbal anaesthesia

- Mechanism unclear
- Cellulose ophthalmic sponge
- Preservative-free 4% lignocaine
- 'Soak time':
  - 1 minute
- Absence epithelial involvement
- Greater comfort
- Quick visual recovery
- Efficacy:
  - Equivalent of drops + LA gel

Table 8.1 Topical anaesthesia preparations

Generic	UK		USA	
	Concentration	Preservative	Concentration	Preservative
Oxybuprocaine	0.4%			
Hydrochloride				
Proxymetacaine	0.5%			
Hydrochloride				
Tetracaine	0.5%		0.5%	Chlorobutanol
Hydrochloride	1%		0.5%	
Tetracaine			0.5%	Benzalkonium
Hydrochloride				
(viscous)				
Proparacaine			0.5% (Alcaine)	Benzalkonium
Hydrochloride			0.5% (Paracaine)	
Lidocaine			0.25%	
			0.25%	Povidone
Lidocaine (gel)			2%	
			2%	
Benoxinate +			4%	Chlorobutanol
fluorescein			4%	

Preservatives

- Alter pH to approximate pH of natural tears—minimize stinging
- Benzalkonium chloride—bactericidal agent
- Disrupt mucous layer tear film—permitting LA direct access to nerve endings

Perioperative considerations

- Patient selection
- Surgeon familiarity with topical anaesthesia
- Standard monitoring includes:
  - ECG, non-invasive blood pressure (BP), pulse oximetry, and respiratory rate monitor
- Intravenous access?
- Supplemental oxygen
- Avoid drape-induced hypercarbia is debatable hypercarbia:
  - Permit venting of exhaled carbon dioxide if draped

- Expose hand:
  - Observe for discomfort and movement
- Comprehensive documentation
- Anaesthesia staff should immediately be available:
  - Intervene for sedation/airway compromise
  - Other adverse events
- Effective communication between all operating room personnel

Conduct of anaesthesia

- Discuss anaesthesia plan with surgeon
- Explanation and reassurance to patient
- Answer patient queries
- Emphasize importance of patient immobility and need to vocalize any discomfort
- Discuss requirement for intraoperative sedation or alternative anaesthesia interventions
- Conduct 'time-out' exercise:
  - Verify correct patient, procedure, site, and any drug allergies
- Instil 1–2 drops aqueous topical:
  - This is done in order to attenuate the sting associated with 5% povidone iodine solution
- Apply 5% povidone iodine solution to cornea
- Cleanse eyelids with iodine solution
- Apply additional topical solution or gel
- Patch or close eye
- Allow sufficient interval for onset anaesthesia

Advantages

- Convenient
- Safe
- Minimal expertise
- Rapid onset
- Painless except simple sting on application
- Avoid complications of needle or cannula-based blocks
- Patient satisfaction

Disadvantages

General
- Incomplete anaesthesia
- Retention of sensory perception, particularly with manipulation
- Visual awareness
- Patients may not have the ability to tolerate bright operating room microscope light
  - Colours may be off-putting
  - Change in light brightness
  - Vague movements
  - Visual alteration during corneal irrigation
- Kinesis (eye movement)
- Unexpected patient movement

Corneal effects
- Decreased tear production
- Epithelial toxicity
- Endothelial toxicity
- Microbial contamination

Systemic effects
- If cocaine used:
  - Hypertension
  - Dysrhythmia
  - Cardiovascular collapse
- Allergic and idiosyncratic responses:
  - Rare allergic reaction to other local anaesthetic agents
  - Proparacaine—contact dermatitis
- Stevens–Johnson syndrome
- Endophthalmitis risk

Sepsis (endophthalmitis) (see Table 8.2)
- Risk of postoperative endophthalmitis:
  - 0.05–0.1%
- Multiple sources including topical preparations (esp. gel)
- Gram-positive organisms
  - *Staphylococcus epidermidis* and *Staphylococcus aureus* (eyelids)
- Prophylaxis aim:
  - Suppress microbial numbers and inhibit microorganism growth

Table 8.2 Sepsis prophylactic measures

Intervention	Efficacy	Evidence-based recommendation
Subconjunctival antibiotics	+/–	C
Lash trimming	–	C
Saline irrigation	–	C
Povidone-iodine	+	B
Topical antibiotics	+/–	C
Irrigation + antibiotic	+/–	C
Heparin	–	C

Povidone iodine
- 5% solution
- Bactericidal
- Must make contact with corneal epithelium
- ❶ Ineffective if applied over gel
- ⚠ Apply iodine solution before gel

Adverse events
- ≤1% cases
- Usually co-existing morbidity especially hypertension and diabetes
- Sedation and airway issues
- Patient movement
- Cough
- 'Vocal local'
  - Unacceptable verbal coaxing of distressed patient
- Reflex autonomic activity
  - Tachycardia and hypertension
- Inadequate anaesthesia
  - Provide effective relief
  - Usually intra-cameral/subconjunctival/sub-Tenon's block/drops

Closed claims data
- 2006 (USA)
  - >20% of Monitored Anesthesia Care claims related to elective eye surgery cases
- 1992 (USA)
  - 30% of eye injury claims related to patient movement

Conclusion

Topical anaesthesia has gained popularity over the last decades for simple routine operations like uncomplicated cataract in selected patients. Topical anaesthesia is usually supplemented with sedation. Sedation carries its own side effects and complications. Although topical anaesthesia is simple and reasonably effective in selected patients and avoids the complications of needle and cannula-based blocks but it does have its own disadvantages.

Further reading

Bhananker SM, Posner KL, Cheney FW et al. Injury and liability associated with monitored anesthesia care. A closed claims analysis. *Anesthesiology*. 2006; 104: 228–234.

Ciulla TA, Starr MB, Masket S. Bacterial endophthalmitis prophylaxis for cataract surgery. An evidence-based update. *Ophthalmology*. 2002; 109(1): 13–24.

Ezra DG, Namibiar A, Allan BD. Supplementary intracameral lidocaine for phacoemulsification under topical anesthesia. A meta-analysis of randomized controlled trials. *Ophthalmology*. 2008; 115(3): 455–87.

Mullin GS, Rubinfeld RS. The antibacterial activity of topical anesthetics. *Cornea*. 1997; 16(6): 662–5.

Page MA, Fraunfelder FW. Safety, efficacy and patient acceptability of lidocaine hydrochloride ophthalmic gel as topical ocular anesthetic for use in ophthalmic procedures. *Clinical Ophthalmology*. 2009; 3: 601–9.

Rosenwasser GO. Complications of topical ocular anesthetics. *Int. Ophth. Clin.* 1989; 29(3): 153–8.

Sharwood PL, Thomas D, Roberts TV. Adverse medical events associated with cataract surgery performed under topical anesthesia. *Clin. & Exp. Ophthalmology*. 2008; 36: 842–6.

Chapter 9

Monitored sedation for ophthalmic surgery

Dr Chin Wui Kin

Dr Benjamin Chang

Introduction

Modern ophthalmic surgery has progressed from an inpatient general anaesthesia procedure to an ambulatory surgery monitored anaesthesia care (MAC) procedure. The majority of eye surgeries, including cataract, anterior segment surgery, oculoplastic, vitreoretinal and strabismus surgery can now, and sometimes are, preferentially performed under regional anaesthesia.

- Sedation during regional anaesthesia for ophthalmic surgery has an important place. The ability to alleviate patient anxiety and increase comfort can improve the overall surgical experience for both patient and surgeon. This chapter will outline the various considerations of monitored sedation during ophthalmic surgery.

Aims of monitored sedation

The primary aim of sedation in surgery is to ensure anxiolysis. Added benefits which may occur are analgesia, amnesia, and somnolence.

There are various factors which determine the type of sedation used:
- Patient factors—age, sex, past medical history, psychological nature, medication history, allergies and anaesthetic history:
  - Ophthalmic patients are usually elderly with multiple medical problems (see 🕮 Chapter 12, Anaesthetic considerations in the elderly, pp. 185–196)
- Procedure factors—duration, complexity, and associated pain:
  - Short procedures, e.g. phacoemulsification cataract surgery, require little sedation; longer procedures, e.g. oculoplastic surgery, may require continuous sedation techniques
- Surgeon factors—preference for light or heavy sedation
- Anaesthetist factors—experience and familiarity with the various sedatives and ophthalmic surgical procedures

Monitored anaesthesia care

- Monitored sedation comes under the broad category of MAC, which can be defined as the provision of a specific anaesthesia service for a diagnostic or therapeutic procedure
- It involves every single aspect of proper anaesthetic management for a patient including:
  - Preoperative assessment
  - Intraoperative management
  - Post-procedure care
- During MAC, the physician will provide the following care:
  - Administration of sedatives, anxiolytics, analgesics, anaesthetic drugs or any other medications as necessary
  - Diagnosis and management of any medical issues intra-procedure
  - Monitoring and support of vital functions
  - Psychological support
    — Ensuring physical comfort
  - Conversion to general anaesthesia when necessary
- MAC involves more than sedation. The practitioner must be prepared to:
  - Assess and manage any physiological derangements and medical problems during the procedure

- Rescue a patient's airway from any sedation or regional anaesthesia-induced compromise (brainstem anaesthesia, intravascular injection of local anaesthetics, etc.)
- Provide general anaesthesia as required by the patient or procedure
- Recover patients post-procedure. This includes:
  — A return to full conscious state
  — Relief of pain
  — Management of any adverse physiological responses
  — Management of side effects from medications

Preoperative assessment

MAC covers the entire spectrum of anaesthesia care from preoperative assessment to postoperative care (see 📖 Chapter 5, Preoperative assessment and preparation, pp. 67–88 & Chapter 22, Patient positioning for eye surgery, pp. 354–66).

- Preoperative assessment is essential for the formulation of a good anaesthetic management plan. Inadequate preparation preoperatively can result in anaesthetic morbidity and mortality
- Purpose of a preoperative assessment:
  - Establishing a doctor–patient relationship
    — Psychologically preparing the patient for surgery
    — Improving patient satisfaction
  - History and examination
  - Laboratory investigations as warranted
  - Risk assessment
  - Optimization for surgery
  - Obtain informed consent
  - Prescription of the anaesthesia care plan

Establishing a doctor–patient relationship

A preoperative visit helps to establish rapport with the patient. The anaesthetist can explain the anaesthetic care plan to the patient and answer any questions related to the care during and after the procedure.

History and examination

A complete medical history should be obtained from the patient. Special attention must be paid to the following areas:

- Cardiovascular system:
  - Patients undergoing ophthalmic surgery are frequently elderly and have hypertension, diabetes or heart disease
    — Specific questions about orthopnoea, exertional dyspnoea, and angina should be asked
    — Seek evidence of ischaemic risk, severe angina, decompensated congestive heart failure, severe valvulopathy, or significant dysrhythmia
- Respiratory system:
  - Enquire specifically about the presence of exertional dyspnoea or dyspnoea at rest
    — Smoking history and any symptoms of an upper respiratory tract infection should be elicited
    — Inability to remain supine may be a relative contraindication to surgery, so seek history of cough, obstructive sleep apnoea, post-nasal drip, orthopnoea, etc.
- Neurologic system:
  - Dementia
  - Ability to communicate
  - Deafness
  - Tremor
- Musculoskeletal system:
  - Patient positioning may need to be modified with significant scoliosis, lumbar or cervical spine pathology, or advanced arthritis

- Endocrine system:
  - Patients should also be asked about their blood sugar control if they have diabetes
- Ophthalmic history:
  - History of severe myopia
  - History of sclera buckle placement
  - Quality of vision in both operative and non-operative eyes
- Previous anaesthesia:
  - A history of previous anaesthesia should be sought
    — Ask for postoperative nausea and vomiting and any other complications
    — Review the previous anaesthetic record and note the type of anaesthesia received and any documented problems such as difficult airway or inability to remain relatively still during surgery
- Drug history and allergy:
  - Review the patient's current medication list
    — Document any drug allergies
    — Note presence of latex allergy
    — Special attention should be paid to the use of any anticoagulation medications
- The anaesthetist is expected to perform a physical examination even if the patient is healthy and without any co-existing medical problems
  - Pay particular attention to the blood pressure, presence of any cardiac arrhythmias and assessment of the oral airway for ease of tracheal intubation
  - If the anaesthetist performs the ophthalmic regional block, particular attention should be given to the surface anatomy and the globe–orbit relationship

Investigations

Investigations are performed only if indicated by the patient's medical condition after a thorough assessment. Routine investigations are of little use.
Consider performing the following investigations:
- ECG:
  - Patients above the age of 60 especially there is a history of cardiac disease, unstable angina, tachycardia, severe bradycardia, new onset irregular pulse, history of hypertension and recent syncope event
- Urea, electrolytes, thyroid panel, haematocrit:
  - History of renal failure, liver disease or malnutrition
  - Medication history that includes diuretics or anti-hypertensive
    — Cachexia
    — Recent history of poor oral intake
    — Recent nausea, emesis or diarrhoea
- Blood glucose
  - Patients who have a history of diabetes or receiving corticosteroids
    — Polydipsia or polyuria
- Coagulation tests
  - History of bleeding disorders
  - Medication history of anticoagulants

Risk assessment and optimization for surgery

After a complete history, physical examination and investigations, an assessment on the risk of anaesthesia and surgery can be made.

- Consider postponing elective surgery if the existing medical condition is not under optimal control. Refer the patient to the appropriate physician for management of the medical condition

Intraoperative management

The objectives of intraoperative care are:
- Monitoring vital signs
- Diagnosis of any medical issues
- Ensuring patient comfort
- Providing anxiolytics, analgesics and other necessary medications
- Creating optimal surgical conditions
- Ensuring rapid return to preoperative state

Monitoring

All patients receiving MAC should be monitored with:
- Electrocardiogram
- Non-invasive blood pressure monitors
- Pulse oximetry
- In addition, the use of capnography and other monitors such as precordial stethoscope or processed electroencephalogram (EEG) bispectral index (BIS), for example, can be considered
- Most importantly, the practitioner must be vigilant and alert to any problem that may arise during the procedure. Constant communication with the patient is vital
- The depth of sedation is best monitored using a tool like the Ramsay's score (see Table 9.1) which is reliable and valid. Clinical observation only allows a rough distinction between adequate, inadequate or over sedation.

Table 9.1 Ramsay's Sedation Scale

Patient is anxious and agitated or restless, or both	1
Patient is cooperative, oriented, and tranquil	2
Patient responds to commands only	3
Patient exhibits brisk response to light glabellar tap or loud auditory stimulus	4
Patient exhibits a sluggish response to light glabellar tap or loud auditory stimulus	5
Patient exhibits no response	6

Techniques

Communication with the patient is important in alleviating anxiety. A preoperative visit to explain the procedure and what to expect during the procedure increases patient's satisfaction. Simple measures like EMLA cream to the dorsum before intravenous (IV) cannulation and the use of a thermal blanket improves patient comfort.
- The key to successful ophthalmic day surgery is titration of fast-acting, short-duration drugs that allow rapid return to baseline function.
- Anxiolytic and analgesic drugs may be necessary to provide comfort to the patient during the procedure. These drugs have the potential

to depress the respiratory system. Provide oxygen to the patient and exercise vigilance in monitoring for any respiratory compromise.

- Oxygen may need to be discontinued during electrocautery for some oculoplastic procedures.

Drugs

Propofol

Propofol (2,6-diisopropylphenol) is a phenolic derivative which is highly lipid soluble. It presents as a white emulsion which contains soya bean oil, egg phosphatide and glycerol.

- Propofol acts by affecting the gamma-aminobutyric acid (GABA) receptors in the central nervous system. It can produce rapid loss of consciousness by the immediate uptake in the central nervous system
- Terminal half-life of propofol is 5–12 hours. Elimination of propofol is dependent on liver metabolism. Conjugated propofol is then excreted in the kidneys
- The side effects of propofol are:
  - Pain on injection
  - Excitatory movements like myoclonus and convulsions
  - Hypotension
  - Depression of the respiratory system and apnoea
- The anaesthetist must be cautious when electing to use propofol for ophthalmic surgery cases. Abruptly altered levels of consciousness induced by onset or offset of propofol can lead to unexpected patient movement. Exaggerated movement during critical portions of ophthalmic surgery can contribute to poor visual outcome
- Propofol can be administered by the following methods:
  - Slow bolus of propofol 0.2–0.5mg/kg can be given before the administration of a regional block
  - Infusion of propofol 0.8–3.0mg/kg/hour can be given throughout the procedure
  - A target-controlled infusion (TCI) with target concentrations of 0.4–1.0mcg/ml can be used
- Consider supplementation with an analgesic drug like fentanyl 50mcg or remifentanil (0.3–1.0mcg/kg) bolus during periods of intense pain or stimulation

Benzodiazepines

Midazolam is a benzodiazepine that is highly lipid soluble. It produces sedation, hypnosis, anxiolysis, and anterograde amnesia by enhancing GABA-mediated inhibition in the central nervous system.

- Midazolam is metabolized in the liver and the subsequent metabolites are eliminated in the urine. It does not produce active metabolites resulting in a rapid recovery and absence of hangover effects. Terminal half-life is 2h
- Midazolam can be administered by the following methods:
  - Boluses of midazolam 0.015–0.3mg/kg but careful titration to achieve the desired effect is required
  - Slow boluses intravenously in 0.5–2mg increments

- Patient controlled sedation where the bolus dose is 0.1mg
  - Intramuscular and nasal administrations although practiced in many countries have been largely abandoned for adult patients
- The reversal agent, flumazenil, may be administered in small incremental doses (up to 0.2–0.4mg) should the patient become excessively sedate

Dexmedetomidine

Dexmedetomidine is a selective and specific agonist of the $\alpha2$ receptors. Presynaptic activation of the $\alpha2$ receptor inhibits the release of nor-adrenaline and modulates the transmission of nociceptive signals.

- Postsynaptic activation of the $\alpha2$ receptors inhibits sympathetic activity. Activation of the $\alpha2$ receptors in the central nervous system results in sedative and analgesic effects
- Dexmedetomidine produces sedation, anxiolysis and analgesic effects with little danger of respiratory depression
- It undergoes liver metabolism with the metabolites excreted in the kidneys. Its elimination half-life is about 2h
- Dexmedetomidine may be associated with paroxysmal patient movement upon stimulation. Movement during critical aspects of ophthalmic surgery may result in poor visual outcome. The use of an auxiliary agent such as a short-acting narcotic or benzodiazepine should be considered
- Unwanted effects of dexmedetomidine:
  - Bradycardia
  - Hypotension
- Be aware of bradycardic effects of dexmedetomidine. Ophthalmic surgery is associated with bradydysrhythmia due to oculo-cardiac reflex
- Dexmedetomidine can be administered by the following method:
  - Loading dose of 1mcg/kg over 10min. Continue with maintenance infusion of 0.2–0.4mcg/kg/hour

Remifentanil

Remifentanil is an ester synthetic opioid that acts mainly on the μ receptors producing sedation and analgesia. It is rapidly hydrolysed by non-specific plasma enzymes resulting in a very rapid offset of activity.

- Remifentanil has small volume of distribution (0.4L/kg) and a high clearance (50ml/kg/min) and hence a very short elimination half-life (3–10min). This makes it suitable to be used as an infusion when a rapid offset is required. Elimination is organ independent
- Unwanted effects:
  - Bradycardia
  - Respiratory depression
  - Nausea and vomiting
- Whilst the rapid abatement of effect of remifentanil confers a modicum of additional safety; when used as the primary agent during MAC for eye surgery, patient awareness and lack of amnesia are not uncommon. Patients should be informed that awareness during surgery is not unusual, and in fact, expected

- Remifentanil can be administered by the following methods:
  - A single slow bolus intravenous dose of 0.3–1.0mcg/kg, about 90s before the regional block or surgical stimulus
  - Infuse of 0.1mcg/kg/min about 5min before the regional block, then reduce to 0.025mcg/kg/min after the block and titrate to effect
  - A single intravenous dose of 0.3–0.5mcg/kg over 30–60s in combination with other agents (such as Propofol 0.05–0.5mg/kg before the block)

Fentanyl
Fentanyl is a phenylpiperidine synthetic opioid which acts predominantly via the μ receptor. It is analgesic drug with little sedative activity at low doses. Fentanyl is highly lipid soluble with a rapid onset and short duration of action at low doses.

- Fentanyl is metabolized in the liver and the metabolites are excreted in the kidneys. The terminal half-life is 3–4h. However, with multiple doses or a prolonged infusion the duration of action is significantly prolonged
- Unwanted side effects:
  - Nausea and vomiting
  - Respiratory depression
- Some ophthalmic surgical procedures are associated with a high incidence of postoperative nausea and emesis. Some patients are also more prone to postoperative nausea and vomiting. Consider minimizing or eliminating the use of opioid analgesics for these patients
- Fentanyl can be administered by the following methods:
  - Bolus doses of 25–50mcg
  - Patient-controlled analgesia (PCA) with a loading dose of 0.7mcg/kg, bolus dose of 0.5mcg and a 5min lockout interval.

Ketamine
Ketamine is a phencyclidine derivative that is an effective sedative/analgesic when used in low doses

- Sedation with ketamine is not associated with respiratory depression
- Unwanted side effects:
  - Secretions
  - Hypertension, tachycardia
  - Confusion, hallucination
  - Rotatory nystagmus and cycloplegia blepharospasm
- These side effects are more typically encountered with larger doses
- Consider premedication with an anticholinergic (carefully in elderly)
- Consider premedication with a benzodiazepine

Etomidate
Etomidate has been used for sedation in patients with severe cardiovascular impairment.

- Side effects make it a less than ideal agent for ophthalmic surgical procedures:
  - Burning upon injection
  - Excitatory movements like myoclonus and convulsions
  - High incidence of nausea and emesis

Complications during monitored sedation

Airway obstruction and apnoea

Airway obstruction can result from over-sedation, obstructive sleep apnoea, and more. The excessive use or idiosyncratic reaction to sedative drugs can lead to a decreased conscious state and unconsciousness. This can lead to upper airway obstruction as the tongue falls back against the posterior pharyngeal wall.

- The sedative drugs can depress the respiratory centre resulting in a slower respiratory rate and even apnoea. This can lead to decreased haemoglobin oxygen saturation and eventually hypoxemia
- The signs of airway obstruction are stridor or stentorous breath sounds, decreased chest movement (which may be masked by ventilatory effort), absence of breath sounds on auscultation, and cyanosis
- Cyanosis and a drop in haemoglobin oxygen saturation are late signs
- Apnoea is detected by monitoring the patient closely for chest movements and breath sounds. The use of capnography to monitor the end tidal CO_2 and plethysmography to monitor chest movement may help to detect apnoea early
- End tidal CO_2 measured via a nasal cannula is a qualitative, not quantatative value. It can be used to assess respiratory rate and re-breathing of expired air
- Airway obstruction and apnoea after ophthalmic regional anaesthesia is a medical emergency and requires immediate management
  - Differential diagnosis includes brainstem anaesthesia, orbital epidural injection, intravascular injection, excessive or idiosyncratic response to sedation, and more
  - Immediately provide 100% oxygen to the patient using a face mask as necessary
  - Relieve the obstruction by providing 'jaw thrust' and 'chin lift'
  - Use an oral airway or nasal airway if obstruction is not relieved by manual manoeuvres
  - If patient is apnoeic, ventilate gently using the bag and mask apparatus
  - Consider supraglottic airway or endotracheal intubation for refractive cases of brainstem anaesthesia induced apnoea
  - Ensure that any infusion of sedative drugs is stopped
- Assist the patient until stable and able to protect own airway. Ensure that the rate and depth of breathing as well as protective reflexes are adequate
- Distinguishing apnoea due to sedation versus central spread of ophthalmic block:
  - Examine the contralateral unblocked eye
  - A mydriatic (dilated) pupil may be indicative of local anaesthetic flow across the optic nerve chiasm to the other eye
  - A miotic (constricted) pupil may be a sign of narcotic overdose

- After the patient arouses, decreased vision or impaired mobility of the contralateral, unblocked eye are pathognomonic for central spread of local anaesthetics
- Administer appropriate reversal agent (flumazenil, naloxone)
- Improvement is indicative of apnoea due to sedatives
- Failure to resolve apnoea bolsters central spread of injected local anaesthetics as causative

Movements

Excessive patient movement during ophthalmic block or eye surgery can contribute to untoward postoperative visual outcome.

- More than 20% of MAC closed claims cases in the ASA (American Society of Anesthesiologists) database occurred with patients undergoing ophthalmic surgery
- The most common causes in these cases were attributed to the eye block and perioperative unwanted patient movement
- The anaesthetist's preoperative assessment should seek to determine if there is an increased likelihood of gross patient movement during eye surgery
- Factors that increase potential for movement include:
  - Cough
  - Post-nasal drip
  - Obstructive sleep apnoea
  - Pathologic anxiety, true severe panic attacks
  - Fluctuating levels of consciousness
  - Re-breathing of carbon dioxide under occluded drapes
- Elective ophthalmic surgery should be postponed until such time that the patient is in optimal condition to remain relatively still during the procedure
- Patients should be made aware of the risks and potential visual ramifications of gross movement during critical parts of ophthalmic surgery
- General anaesthesia is not often a suitable option as it may be associated with untoward consequences as well for example:
  - The patient with a cough is at increased risk for laryngospasm and bronchospasm
  - The patient with a cough is at increased risk of bucking and straining upon emergence from general anaesthesia. The subsequent increase in intra-ocular pressure can damage the operated eye
  - A patient with orthopnoea due to chronic obstructive pulmonary disease may require prolonged postoperative intubation
- Deliberate patient selection and judicious choice of type of anaesthetic is requisite in order to provide optimal anaesthesia care

Oculo-cardiac reflex

The anaesthetist must be wary of the oculo-cardiac reflex (OCR) and be ready to intervene promptly as needed (see 📖 Oculo-cardiac reflex, p. 44)

- The OCR can occur during:
  - Administration of regional anaesthesia
  - Ophthalmic surgery under general anaesthesia
  - Squint surgery presents greatest risk

- Prevention:
  - Preoperative anticholinergics have dubious effectiveness
  - Tachycardia secondary to anticholinergics may induce myocardial ischemia and have greater adverse consequence than transient OCR-induced bradycardia
- Treatment:
  - Stop the causative stimulus (block, pressure on the globe, pulling of an extra-ocular muscle)
  - Wait until restoration of normal rate and rhythm. The OCR displays tachyphylaxis; the response wanes with repeated elicitation
  - Consider anticholinergics for refractive cases or if asystole

Hypotension

Sedative agents can cause a drop in blood pressure. Propofol causes a drop in systemic vascular resistance and depresses cardiac output. Dexmedetomidine acts via the $\alpha2$ receptor to inhibit vasomotor response.

- Hypotension can be significant, especially with propofol. Corrective steps should be taken including:
  - Fluid challenge—start with a crystalloid solution like Ringer's lactate or normal saline. Consider administering 3–5ml/kg bolus.
  - Consider the use of a vasopressor like ephedrine or phenylephrine. Titrate with 3–6mg of ephedrine bolus or 50–100mcg of phenylephrine.

Postoperative care

There is considerable international variation in practice regarding the need for stage I recovery room monitoring for patients who have undergone ophthalmic surgery via MAC. In some areas, provided that the patient is sufficiently stable, discharge directly to stage II recovery is the norm. In those venues in which monitoring in the postanaesthesia care unit (PACU) are provided, it should be located close to the operating theatres and staffed by adequately trained nurses.

- Patients should be monitored with a pulse oximeter, ECG, and non-invasive blood pressure monitor
- The PACU nurse should monitor and record the pulse rate, oxygen saturation, blood pressure and respiratory rate every 5min for an appropriate duration of time
- The level of consciousness, pain score and temperature may also be recorded
- Consider providing supplemental oxygen if patient is heavily sedated or has needs otherwise
- Consider convection air warming if the ambient temperature is cold
- Discharge criteria may include:
  - Consciousness (awake, alert and orientated)
  - Stable vital signs
  - Adequate respiration
  - Minimal or no pain
    — No nausea or vomiting
  - No obvious surgical complication (bleeding)
- All patients who have received sedation should be accompanied home by a family member

Complications in PACU

Airway obstruction

Airway obstruction may occur in the semiconscious patient in PACU. This is due to the tongue falling back against the posterior pharynx. Look out for absent breath sounds and paradoxical movements of the chest.

- Provide supplemental oxygen for patients with airway obstruction. Use the jaw-thrust and head tilt manoeuvre when not contraindicated in order to open the airway.
- Consider the use of an oral or nasal airway
- Consider narcotic and benzodiazepine antagonist agents

Hypoventilation

Observe for excessive somnolence, slow respiratory rate or laboured breathing. Hypoventilation is usually due to the effects of the sedative drugs on the respiratory system.

- Marked hypoventilation may require urgent treatment:
  - Assist ventilation using a bag and mask device with supplemental oxygen
  - Consider treating the cause by reversing the effect of the sedative drugs
  - Reverse the effects of opioid using incremental doses of naloxone (fractional dosing to 0.04mg)
  - Reverse the effects of benzodiazepines by using flumazenil (start with up to 0.2mg and then 0.1mg increments)

Hypoxia

Hypoxia is common and may result from excessive sedation and hypoventilation. Look out for restlessness, obtundation, tachycardia or bradycardia and hypotension. The use of a pulse oximeter should facilitate early detection.

- Hypoxia is treated by providing supplemental oxygen (30–40%). If hypoxemia is severe or persistent, apply 100% oxygen via a non-re-breathing mask. Look for the cause and treat the cause. Mechanical ventilation may be required

Nausea and vomiting

Retching, nausea, and emesis are all associated with specific ophthalmic surgical procedures (see 📖 Regional anaesthesia, p. 160, Syndromes associated with strabismus, p. 261 and Postoperative management, p. 267).

- Patients at greatest risk include:
  - Strabismus surgery
  - Oculoplastic surgery
  - Elevated post-surgical intra-ocular pressure
  - Those with a history of postoperative nausea and vomiting
  - Those with history of motion sickness
  - Youth > elderly
  - Non smokers > smokers
- Consider prophylactic administration of combination therapy antiemetics for those patients at greatest risk

Conclusion

The main objectives of monitored sedation for ophthalmic surgery are safety, anxiolysis, amnesia, and analgesia. Ensuring patient comfort and safety is also of paramount importance. Patients should be vigilantly monitored for their vital signs and breathing. MAC stands for Maximal Anaesthetist Concern, not Minimal Anaesthesia Care! The use of ECG, pulse oximetry, non-invasive blood pressure monitor and capnography (or precordial stethoscope) is recommended. Patients undergoing monitored sedation should be managed as though they will be receiving general anaesthesia. They should undergo a proper preoperative assessment and adhere to appropriate fasting guidelines.

There are a number of sedative drug options, each with different pharmacokinetic and pharmacodynamic variables. The practitioner should tailor their use to the specific patient, procedure, surgeon, venue, etc.

Complications such as brainstem anaesthesia, intravascular injection of local anaesthetics, airway obstruction, apnoea, dysrhythmias, hyper- or hypotension, retching and nausea/emesis can occur and the anaesthetist must monitor for them vigilantly. Urgent resuscitation steps must be taken immediately as indicated.

Further reading

Greenhalgh DL, Kumar CM. Sedation during ophthalmic surgery. *European Journal of Anaesthesiology*. 2008; 25: 701–7.

Distinguishing monitored anesthesia care ('MAC') from moderate sedation/analgesia (conscious sedation). American Society of Anesthesiologists.http://www.asahq.org/publicationsAndServices/standards/35.pdf, accessed 29 March 2011.

Position on monitored anesthesia care. American Society of Anesthesiologists.http://www.asahq.org/publicationsAndServices/standards/23.pdf, accessed 29 March 2011.

Guidance on the provision of ophthalmic anaesthesia services. Royal College of Anaesthetists. http://www.rcoa.ac.uk/docs/GPAS-Ophth.pdf, accessed 29 March 2011.

Chapter 10

Anaesthesia for oculoplastic surgical procedures

Dr Waleed Riad Imtiaz

Mr Imtiaz A. Chaudhry

Introduction

The focus of this chapter is to acquaint the reader with up-to-date anaesthetic consideration for the safe and optimal performance of the majority of procedures in the oculoplastic subspecialty.

Trauma, congenital defects, changes associated with the ageing process, and tumours affecting the eyelids as well as the tissues and bones surrounding the eyes can cause visual disturbance, cosmetic disfigurement, and significant discomfort.

Typical conditions frequently treated by an oculoplastic surgeon may include:
- Age-related cosmetic deformities
- Eyelid, canalicular and orbital trauma
- Eyelid/orbital tumours
- Correction of traumatic scarring
- Enucleation or evisceration
- Reconstruction of an anophthalmic socket

Anatomical considerations

Understanding the anatomy of the eyelids and the lacrimal apparatus is essential for correct placement of local anaesthetic (LA) and to avoid damage to the globe or the tear drainage system.

The eyelids and structures around the eyes are critical for vision and facial appearance. There are several anatomic relations to consider when performing peri-ocular injections.

- The eyelids are about 2–3mm in thickness depending on the age of the patient
- The height of the superior tarsal plate ranges between 10–14mm while the height of the lower tarsal plate ranges between 3–4mm
- In the upper eyelid, the levator aponeurosis attaches to the tarsal plate on the anterior surface, and the Muller muscle inserts on the superior edge of the tarsus
- Equivalent structures exist in the lower eyelid, composed of the capsulopalpebral fascia and the inferior tarsal muscle
- The orbital septum separates the eyelid fat pads posteriorly from the anterior lamella
- The main anterior blood supply of the upper eyelid is divided between two branches of the palpebral vessels:
  - The superior marginal artery lies 2mm from the eyelid margin
  - The peripheral arcade is found at the superior edge of the tarsus between the levator aponeurosis and Muller muscle
- The lower eyelid is supplied by the inferior marginal artery
- Tears are produced by the lacrimal gland then distributed over the surface of the eye by blinking
- They drain during the relaxation phase of blinking via superior and inferior lacrimal puncta (near the medial ends of upper and lower lid margins) into the lacrimal sac through the lacrimal canaliculi
- The lacrimal sac is situated in the lacrimal fossa in the anterior part of the medial wall of the orbit
- Tears pass through the nasolacrimal duct which connects the inferior end of the lacrimal sac to the inferior meatus of the nose
- The lacrimal drainage system receives its sensory and autonomic innervations through zygomaticotemporal and lacrimal nerves

Preoperative evaluation

Preoperative planning (see 📖 Goals of preoperative assessment, p. 68) can help reduce the operative time and decrease potential complications of oculoplastic surgery.

- Information about past medical, surgical, medication, and family history can modify the anaesthetic plan:
  - For instance, a history of failure of previous dacryocystorhinostomy (DCR) may affect the choice of surgical and anaesthetic techniques
  - Surgery may be contraindicated in the anticoagulated patient
- Physical examination should include evaluation of the surface anatomy and lacrimal system for presence of inflammation and/or a mucocoele over the medial canthal area. Routine laboratory screening is not warranted (see 📖 Laboratory studies, p. 72)
- Patients receiving anticoagulant medications are of special concern
- Unlike other types of ophthalmic surgery, anticoagulation may be an absolute contraindication to oculoplastic surgery as orbital or lid haemorrhage could affect cosmetic and/or functional outcome
- In those patients at higher risk for weaning from anticoagulants, the surgeon, internist/cardiologist, and patient should agree on a course of action (see 📖 Anticoagulant therapy and ophthalmic surgery, p. 79)

Since most of the oculoplastic procedures are not urgent, preoperative optimization of comorbidities is indicated.

Premedication

The practice of premedication varies worldwide based on the anaesthetist's experience and preference, availability of medication, and patient's general condition.

For patients undergoing general anaesthesia (GA), our current practice is to use oral benzodiazepine (i.e. lorazepam) and H_2 receptor antagonist the night before and at the morning of surgery for adults. Practices vary.

Oral/intramuscular(IM)/intranasal midazolam is commonly used for children in addition to oral/rectal analgesics such as paracetamol or non-steroidal anti-inflammatory drugs (NSAIDs). Various options exist.

General anaesthesia

The anaesthetic plan should be tailored to the individual patient. GA is the technique of choice for:

- Bony orbital procedures
- Prolonged procedures
- Moderate or severe trauma
- Gross localized infection
- Paediatric patients
- Patients with uncontrolled tremors
- Severe language or communication barriers
- True allergy to LA solutions
- Patient or surgeon request

Patients who have had a previous complication or suboptimal experience with ophthalmic regional blockade should be considered for GA.

An established fasting guideline is followed.

Considerations for day-case surgery are the same as for other ocular procedures, so drugs that are rapidly metabolized and eliminated are preferable.

- This typically includes propofol induction, fentanyl or remifentanil, NSAIDs as analgesics and short- or intermediate-acting muscle relaxants:
  - Neuromuscular blocking agents may have residual effects
  - Muscle relaxant reversal agents may be problematic, so consider avoiding the use of muscle relaxants

Children can be induced by either an inhalational or intravenous technique; selection of the technique depends on the child's cooperation, ease of venepuncture, anaesthetists' preference and the clinical situation (see 🕮 Chapter 13, Anaesthesia for paediatric ophthalmic surgery, pp. 197–222).

The choice between supraglottic devices and standard endotracheal intubation (ETT) depends on the duration and the nature of the procedure.

- An oral ETT (Rae) angles away from the surgical field as this can be readily anchored to the chin, preventing inadvertent endobronchial intubation by pressure from drapes, surgeons, assistants etc.
- A flexible LMA allows the surgeon to move the device's shank such that mucosal tissue is more easily accessible for harvesting
- Special attention should be paid to patients presenting for ectropion repair secondary to a severe burn:
  - Thermal injury and subsequent scarring may lead to difficult airway management due to skin contracture and internal airway damage
  - If patient presents within 120 days following the thermal injury, a massive release of potassium could occur if suxamethonium is used to facilitate intubation

Anaesthesia is maintained with a standard GA technique with low blood-gas solubility inhalational agent or total intravenous anesthesia (TIVA) infusion.

The oculoplastic surgeon may infiltrate the incision site with 2% lidocaine with 1:100,000 epinephrine to minimize intraoperative bleeding. However, the anaesthetist should be made aware as absorption of epinephrine into the systemic circulation may lead to serious complications such as severe hypertension, myocardial infarction, ventricular fibrillation, pulmonary oedema, cerebral haemorrhage, and cardiac arrest.

Patients suitable for day-case surgery should be 'street fit' postoperatively as early as possible.

Regional anaesthesia

Advantages of regional anaesthesia (RA) compared with GA for oculo-plastic procedures include:
- Reduction in operating room turnover time
- Potentially lower incidence of nausea and vomiting
- Reduced need for postoperative narcotics
- Earlier discharge

Combinations of analgesics and sedative agents are widely used with oculoplastic LA techniques (see ⬚ Chapter 9, Monitored sedation for ophthalmic surgery, pp. 135–152). Various local anaesthetic agents, concentrations, and combinations have been advocated for use in oculoplastic surgical procedures (see ⬚ Chapter 4, Pharmacology for ophthalmic local anaesthesia, pp. 53–66).

- Lidocaine 1–2% can be administered as the sole LA with or without epinephrine (1:100 000 or 1:200 000)
- The effects of lidocaine may start working within minutes of injection and can last up to 2–3h when administered with epinephrine
- Epinephrine may be systemically absorbed, resulting in tachydysrhythmia and thus may be relatively contraindicated
- Bupivacaine 0.25–0.75% can be administered alone or in combination with lidocaine to prolong the effect of local anaesthesia for up to 6h
- There are numerous LAs available for local infiltration
- Shorter-acting agents are often preferable as prolonged postoperative orbicularis weakness and lagophthalmos may result from use of longer-acting LAs

Pain upon injection local anaesthetic agent is related to low pH and rapidity of slow, incremental infiltration
- Addition of sodium bicarbonate 7.5% to increase the pH of the injectate
- Topical skin anaesthetic agents such as lidocaine, EMLA cream, synera patch etc.

Technique of eyelid anaesthetic infiltration

0.5–1.5in, 27–30 gauge needles are commonly used for the infiltration of anaesthetic agent depending on the depth of the peri-ocular blockade needed. Local anaesthesia should be administered slowly and in continuous advancing fashion, causing the tissue ahead of the needle path to balloon.

- While injecting the eyelids, tissue finger traction allows the area being injected to be clearly visualized
- Positioning the non-injecting hand on the forehead or cheek may allow for better stability
- Needle can penetrate the thin and delicate upper eyelid
- An oculopharyngeal reflex may be triggered by periocular injection:
  - Often manifests as involuntary sneezing
  - Time should be given for the sneezing to abate, after which the physician can proceed with the anaesthetic injection
  - A sneeze reflex (and/or involuntary myoclonic movements) may also occur after propofol sedation
  - Unexpected movement from sneezing can result in needle injury to the globe and peri-orbital haematoma which may lead to postponement of the surgery
  - Administration of small dose of narcotic (i.e. fentanyl, alfentanil, remifentanil) may suppress the reflex
- If the globe moves in the direction of the advancing needle or restriction of advancement is noted during injection, the injection should be abandoned
- A subconjuctival injection of LA can create iatrogenic chemosis and pupillary peaking or dilation if the anaesthetic contains epinephrine

Fire risks

Safe patient care may necessitate the use of oxygen. A review of closed claims MAC cases over a ten-year period in the US found that almost one in five legal settlements were attributable to patient burns.

Three factors must be present for a fire to occur in the operating room: a source of ignition, a fuel source, and an enriched oxygen environment. Means to lessen the likelihood of fire include:

- Use the lowest concentration and flow of oxygen (or substitute with air or use oxygen only on standby)
- Establish an impermeable barrier between the patient's nares/mouth and the surgical field
- Use active high-flow suction proximate to the patient's airway to decrease peripheral oxygen flow
- Inform the surgical staff that oxygen is in use
- Remind the surgeon to give notice if cautery will be used

Anaesthesia for common oculoplastic procedures

Nasolacrimal drainage procedures

Tear drainage abnormalities are functional or anatomical. Functional failure may be due to disturbance in the lacrimal pump secondary to facial palsy, laxity of the eyelids, feeble orbicularis muscle or displaced punctum. Anatomical obstruction may be congenital or acquired.

- Probing, nasolacrimal intubation and balloon catheter dilatation are some of the treatment choices in congenital anatomical obstruction. However, dacryocystorhinostomy (DCR) is used only in the presence of epiphora (watery eyes) in the face of stenotic or complete lacrimal system obstruction
- Subclinical chronic inflammation of the nasolacrimal sac (dacryocystitis) followed by fibrosis without any precipitating factor may result in primary acquired nasolacrimal duct obstruction

Dacrcryocystorhinostomy

This may be performed either transdermal, nasal or canalicular route.

- In the external DCR, a direct fistula from lacrimal sac to the nasal space is created as an alternative pathway to enable unobstructed drainage of lacrimal system secretions:
  - In this procedure, a large bony rhinostomy is made through maxillary bone and thin lacrimal bone between the lacrimal sac and middle meatus of the nose
  - The lacrimal sac and nasal mucosa are approached through the skin incision
  - Disadvantages of the external DCR may include intraoperative haemorrhage, canalicular stenosis from manipulation and intubation, corneal abrasion, facial scarring, and possible disruption of the medial canthal ligaments with resultant lacrimal pump dysfunction
- With the recent advances in the functional endoscopic sinus surgery, endoscopic nasal DCR has gained in popularity:
  - The development of mini-endoscopes has enabled endoscopy of the lacrimal drainage system via the lacrimal puncta to visualize the exact site of stenosis
  - The technique involves localization of the medial wall of the lacrimal sac through placement of a lacrimal probe or retinal light either through the lacrimal system or transcanalicular followed by endoscopic incision of the nasal mucosa and osteotomy by fracturing the thin lacrimal bone under endoscope guidance
  - Laser may be used for ablation of the nasal mucosa and cutting of the bone. This is followed by incision of the medial wall lacrimal sac
  - Mitomycin-C may also be used to inhibit fibroblast proliferation to try to prevent osteotomy closure. This technique results in less intraoperative bleeding, improved cosmetic appearance, better postoperative course and preservation of the pump function of the nasolacrimal system

General anaesthesia for DCR

- For DCR under general anaesthesia, endotracheal intubation and throat pack can protect the patient's airway against blood aspiration
- Insertion of a nasal pack soaked with decongestant agents may minimize intraoperative bleeding originating from the nasal cavity. It may also improve surgical field visualization
- Other measures such as head-up position, administration of hypotensive anaesthetic agents, and infiltration of admixtures of lidocaine/epinephrine in the nasal mucosa can further reduce intraoperative bleeding
- Although deep extubation is not routinely recommended due to potential aspiration of blood, a smooth extubation is nonetheless warranted as coughing and straining could increase nasal bleeding

Regional anaesthesia for DCR

Regional anaesthesia for DCR involves blockade of infratrochlear, infraorbital and anterior ethmoidal nerves either by separate injections or by local infiltration along with intranasal injection and packing.

The authors' preferred technique is topical anaesthesia of the eye with oxybuprocaine hydrogen chloride (HCL) 0.4% and tetracaine HCL 1% followed by povidone iodine eye drops 5%. This is followed with medial peribulbar block with a mixture of bupivacaine 0.5% and lidocaine 2% with 5IU/ml hyaluronidase injected between the caruncle and medial canthus to a depth of 1.25cm through a sharp needle. The nostril on the operated side sprayed with 4% lidocaine followed by packing with xylometazoline 0.1%.

Blepharoplasty, entropion, and ectropion

These procedures may be of prolonged duration and are often performed on elderly patients with multiple comorbidities.

In many cases, upper and lower lid blepharoplasty, fat pad repositioning, ptosis correction, tumour removal and reconstruction, and entropion and ectropion repair can be performed on an outpatient basis without GA, using minimal to moderate sedation. The goal should be an awake but relaxed patient.

Upper and lower eyelid blepharoplasty may be indicated for the presence of excess skin and/or orbital fat. Preoperative evaluation should include a thorough medical and ophthalmic history, along with vision check. Symptoms of pre-existing dry eye should be elicited preoperatively, as they directly correlate with postoperative complications.

For blepharoplasty of the upper eyelid, approximately 2ml of LA is infiltrated subcutaneously in several locations in each upper eyelid using 27 or 30 gauge needle prior to preparation. Most oculoplastic surgeons prefer to use lidocaine 2% with 1:100,000 epinephrine.

About 5–10min are usually enough for the maximal vasoconstrictive effects of epinephrine and the skin incision can begin.

Complications of blepharoplasty include retrobulbar haematoma, lower eyelid malposition, dry eye, and may require revision surgery. Local anaesthesia during blepharoplasty can block the optic nerve, ciliary ganglion, and extraocular muscle nerves. Local anaesthesia should be injected judiciously during orbital fat removal to avoid associated complications. Transient bilateral visual impairment with external and internal ophthalmoplegia after blepharoplasty under local anaesthesia has been reported. Blindness following cosmetic blepharoplasty can rarely occur.

Ptosis surgery

Uncorrected ptosis may interfere with a child's development of normal binocular vision.

Ptosis repair surgery is usually performed under RA in adults but GA is used in paediatric cases. Patient cooperation is needed to allow estimation of surgical extent preoperatively and for intraoperative assessment of lid positioning.

- Benzodiazepines administered prior to surgery may exacerbate the degree of ptosis resulting in a surgical overcorrection
- Low-volume LA with epinephrine is injected into the upper eyelid as diffusion of epinephrine posteriorly can activate the sympathetically innervated Muller muscle and result in up to 2mm of transient eyelid retraction. Accordingly, inadequate height correction and residual postoperative ptosis may occur. Conversely, diffusion of the anaesthetic posterior to the orbital septum may inactivate or cause temporary paralysis of the levator muscle, making eyelid height adjustments using patient cooperation impossible

Lid haematoma following LA infiltration may warrant postponement of surgery. Pressure should be immediately applied for 1–2min until bleeding stops.

Peri-ocular and orbital trauma

Trauma to the orbital region may result in ocular, peri-ocular soft tissue, and head injuries (see 📖 Epidemiology of traumatic eye injuries, pp. 298–300). The mechanism of orbital injury is important in the evaluation of the patient; low-velocity impact may produce injuries limited to local areas. High-velocity trauma may be associated with soft tissue and skeletal injuries. Physical examination should include a complete eye examination, position of the globe, extra-ocular motility, and associated soft tissue injuries including the evaluation of nasolacrimal system. Although simple peri-ocular soft tissue injuries can be repaired under local anaesthesia, complex peri-ocular injuries, ocular trauma, and most orbital fractures need to be repaired under GA. Children, uncooperative adults, and extensive injuries usually are best repaired under GA. If the injury is localized or the patient represents a significant anaesthetic risk, local anaesthesia along with intravenous sedation while being monitored can be used providing they have met the usual standards for fasting.

Enucleation, evisceration, and exenteration

Enucleation is a procedure in which the globe is removed intact.
- Current indications for enucleation include suspected or known malignancy, blind painful eye, following severe traumatic rupture, or to improve the appearance of severely disfigured eye
- Enucleation in the setting of trauma can be significantly more challenging because of acute oedema of scattered uveal tissue
- Enucleation may be performed under GA or rarely under RA in selected patients. Choice is based on patient, surgeon, anaesthetists' preferences; patient's medical condition, and ocular status

GA can be augmented with an intra- or extraconal injection. This offers several benefits:
- Decreased need of GA agents
- Potential earlier emergence from GA
- Postoperative pain relief
- Epinephrine-containing LA may decrease local bleeding, facilitating surgery

In patients suspected of intra-ocular malignancy and children having retinoblastoma, minimal manipulation of the globe is advised during the enucleation procedure.

Evisceration involves removal of all of the uveal contents and preservation of the scleral shell which is still attached to all the rectus muscles. The main advantages of evisceration over enucleation in the absence of any intra-ocular malignancy are:
- Simple, with less orbital manipulation
- Quicker, less invasive than enucleation
- Possible superior cosmetic rehabilitation of the anophthalmic socket

Evisceration may be performed under GA or RA. Nerve blocks include intra- or extraconal injection, lid anaesthesia via frontal nerve block and infiltration along the infra-orbital nerve over the inferior orbital rim.

Orbital exenteration consists of removal of the entire orbit and its contents, including orbital fat, conjunctival sac, globe, and the eyelids.

It is used to treat a life-threatening malignancy unresponsive to other treatment.

GA is preferred for exenteration with LA infiltration to provide haemostasis and postoperative comfort. Procedure time may be prolonged and blood loss may be significant.

Neurolytic injections

Debilitating ocular pain poses a significant challenge to the ophthalmologist. When the pain is intractable and the eye has very poor vision and is disfigured, surgical removal of the eye has traditionally been the definitive treatment of choice. Because many patients are uncomfortable psychologically with removal of their eyes, and other patients are not good surgical candidates, an alternative to enucleation is sometimes warranted. Retrobulbar injection of a neurolytic substance such as absolute alcohol, phenol 6.7% and chlorpromazine can often induce long-lasting anaesthesia for a blind painful eye. The neurolytic agent should be deposited near the nerve, therefore peribulbar and/or sub-Tenon's anaesthesia cannot be used. The loss of an eye and associated disfigurement may decrease one's confidence and impair self-image. When removal of an eye is necessary, state-of-the-art prosthetic implants should be used to restore the natural look and motion of the prosthetic eye.

Orbital inflammatory diseases

Graves' ophthalmopathy may range from mild eyelid retraction to a dev-astating process that involves the entire orbit and culminates in gross ocular congestion, massive proptosis, and even blindness. Whether the ophthalmopathy is mild or severe, patients are managed on an individual basis according to the predominant clinical findings, which may include congestion, myopathy, lid retraction, proptosis, and optic neuropathy. The process usually becomes quiescent after 6 months to 3 years; however, the changes caused by fibrosis (lid retraction and ocular muscle enlarge-ment) are permanent.

The cornerstone of surgical treatment for severe cases is bony orbital decompression. These patients may require correction of their retracted eyelids in the form of recession.

To avoid the occurrence of thyrotoxic crisis, GA could be offered only after control of the disease.

Conclusion

Careful anaesthetic plan is needed for oculoplastic surgical procedures. The type of anaesthesia employed depends on the patient's condition, surgical procedures, patient's preference, and surgeon's preference. Local anaesthesia has a particular place in certain oculoplastic procedures.

Further reading

Burroughs JR, Soparkar CN, Patrinely JR, Kersten RC, Kulwin DR, Lowe CL. Monitored anesthesia care for enucleations and eviscerations. *Ophthalmology.* 2003; 110: 311–13.

Calenda E, Retout A, Muraine M. Peribulbar anesthesia for peroperative and postoperative pain control in eye enucleation or evisceration: 31 cases. *J. Fr. Ophtalmol.* 1999; 22: 426–30.

Chen WP. Enucleation, evisceration, and exenteration. In McCord CD Jr, Tanenbaum M, Nunery WR (eds), *Oculoplastic surgery*, 3rd edn. New York: Raven Press, 1995; pp. 581–608.

Ciftci F, Pocan S, Karadayi K, Gulecek O. Local versus general anesthesia for external dacryocystorhinostomy in young patients. *Ophthal. Plast. Reconstr. Surg.* 2005; 21: 201–6.

Kumar CM, Dowd TC, Hawthorne M. Retrobulbar alcohol injection for orbital pain relief under difficult circumstances: a case report. *Ann. Acad. Med. Singapore.* 2006; 35: 260–5.

Merbs SL. Management of a blind painful eye. *Ophthalmol. Clin. North Am.* 2006; 19: 287–92.

Moody BR, Holds JB. Anesthesia for office-based oculoplastic surgery. *Dermatol. Surg.* 2005; 31: 766–9.

Scott IU, Mccabe CM, Flynn HW, Lemus DR, Schiffman JC, Reynolds DS, Pereira MB, Belfort A, Gayer S. Local anesthesia with intravenous sedation for surgical repair of selected open globe injuries. *Am. J. Ophthalmol.* 2002; 134: 707–11.

Vagefi MR, Lin CC, McCann JD, Anderson RL. Local anesthesia in oculoplastic surgery: precautions and pitfalls. *Arch. Facial Plast. Surg.* 2008; 10: 246–9.

Chapter 11

General anaesthesia for adult ophthalmic surgery

Dr Kathryn E. McGoldrick

Dr Edwin Xavier Vicioso

Introduction

The success or failure of ophthalmic surgery, although multifactorial, is inextricably linked to the degree of skill demonstrated by the anaesthetist.

Anaesthetic objectives for ophthalmic surgery include:

- Safety
- Akinesia
- Satisfactory analgesia
- Avoidance or obtundation of the oculo-cardiac reflex
- Prevention of intra-ocular hypertension
- Awareness of potential interactions between ophthalmic drugs and anaesthetic agents

Other exigencies include an appreciation of the anaesthetic implications intrinsic to delicate ocular procedures, including the necessity for a faultlessly smooth induction, maintenance, and emergence from anaesthesia. Indeed, closed claims analysis (American Society of Anesthesiologists) disclosed that 30% of settled eye injury claims related to anaesthetic management were associated with intraoperative patient movement and blindness resulted in all instances.

Moreover, safety issues are intensified by the logistic necessity for the anaesthetist to be positioned at a substantial distance from the patient's face, thus impeding or preventing direct access to the airway. Therefore, it is palpably obvious that clear and effective communication between the anaesthetist and the ophthalmologist is mandatory for optimal patient outcomes.

Patients with eye conditions requiring surgery are often at the extremes of age, ranging from tiny fragile infants with retinopathy of prematurity to nonagenarian or even centenarians with submacular haemorrhage or retinal detachment. Not uncommonly these individuals have complicated associated systemic or metabolic diseases. Moreover, the ageing of the population, especially in developed nations, is pervasive, unprecedented, and profound. Currently, approximately 15% of the population in the US is ≥65 years. The challenges of caring skilfully for an ageing population with extensive comorbidities undergoing technically demanding ophthalmic procedures mandate anaesthetic expertise.

Indications for general anaesthesia

Numerous factors influence the selection of anaesthetic technique for ophthalmic surgery. Although regional and topical techniques have gained impressive popularity recently for selected routine procedures, it is imperative to understand the critical role that GA has in the care of certain ophthalmic patients.

GA is often the method of choice for:
• Children
• Individuals with learning difficulties
• Demented or psychologically unstable patients
• Boney oculoplastic procedures and removal of infected scleral buckles
• Surgery of prolonged duration
• Patients with very high myopia, where a perforating injury from peribulbar or retrobulbar block is feared
• Severely claustrophobic patients
• Deafness
• Those with a language barrier
• Parkinson's disease with severe head tremor, and severe arthritis
• Orthopnoea that limits the patient's ability to lie flat and remain motionless during surgery

It is also the favoured approach for those with suspected or apparent open-globe injuries, although recent literature supports the use of regional eye blocks in selected patients with open-eye trauma.
• Gayer and colleagues explored methods to safely block patients with certain limited open-globe injuries. They repaired 220 disrupted eyes with RA during a 4-year interval at Bascom Palmer Eye Institute. The eyes selected tended to have smaller, more anterior wounds than those repaired with GA, and the injuries were often the result of dehiscence of cataract or corneal transplant incisions. Notably, combined topical analgesia and sedation for selected patients with open-eye injuries has also been reported.

The anticipated duration of the procedure must also be considered, because few geriatric patients having RA can remain comfortable on a narrow, hard operating table for much longer than 3h.

Although GA eliminates the hazards of peribulbar or retrobulbar haemorrhage, globe perforation, myotoxicity, and brainstem anaesthesia, this choice of GA may be associated with:
• Greater likelihood of postoperative nausea and vomiting
• Airway complications
• Post-surgical ophthalmic complications due to valsalva or bucking upon extubation

Accordingly, the risks, benefits, and alternatives of all anaesthetic options must be explained clearly to the patient, with the selection determined after discussion between patient, surgeon, and anaesthetist.

Preoperative evaluation

Special issues must be considered during the preoperative evaluation of geriatric patients (see 📖 Recovery, p. 195). There is enormous inter-individual variation in terms of the ageing process, and chronological age is a poor surrogate for fitness or frailty. Nonetheless, even 'normal' ageing results in changes in cardiac, respiratory, neurologic, and renal physiology that are associated with reduced functional reserve and ability to compensate for physiologic stress. Superimposed on these changes is the fact that elderly patients frequently take multiple medications that can alter homeostatic mechanisms.

Preoperative testing (see 📖 Guidelines for preoperative care, pp. 72–73)

- Laboratory testing should be selective, based on abnormalities identified from the patient's history and physical examination, rather than consisting of a routine battery of tests
- Routine testing is expensive, and the positive predictive value of abnormal findings on generic, routine screening is limited
- The preoperative period is not the time to screen for asymptomatic disease, and positive results on screening tests have modest impact on patient care
- Moreover, false positives occur, and failure to follow-up on these 'abnormalities' may expose the clinician to litigation
- Because age itself confers only slight incremental risk in the absence of co-existing disease, most risk-stratification indices have focused on specific diseases

Preoperative considerations for patients with cardiac disease

Structural changes occur in the cardiovascular system as patients age, and there is a decline in autonomic responsiveness/control that can result in haemodynamic instability. Superimposition of such conditions as angina or valvular heart disease can further impede cardiovascular performance, especially in the perioperative period.

According to the 2007 American College of Cardiology/American Heart Association (ACC/AHA) Guidelines, the goal of the preoperative evaluation should be the identification of major predictors of cardiac risk such as:

- Unstable coronary syndromes
- Unstable angina
- Myocardial infarction (MI) <30 days ago
- Decompensated congestive heart failure (CHF)
- Severe valvular disease
- Arrhythmias, such as high degree atrioventricular block, symptomatic ventricular arrhythmias, supraventricular tachycardia with uncontrolled ventricular rate

These patients with active cardiac conditions have a prohibitive rate of perioperative morbidity and mortality, and are inappropriate candidates for elective outpatient surgery. They deserve the benefit of further cardiology consultation and optimization.

The Revised Cardiac Risk Index of Lee and colleagues was the result of an important study of 4315 patients older than 50 years of age who were having non-cardiac elective surgery. Six independent perioperative risk factors were identified:

- High-risk surgery
- Intraperitoneal
- Intrathoracic
- Suprainguinal vascular
- A history of ischemic heart disease
- CHF
- Cerebrovascular disease
- Preoperative treatment with insulin
- Serum creatinine >2.0mg/dL

The authors specifically note, however, that this index is of uncertain generalizability in lower-risk populations, such as those having minor procedures.

The ACC/AHA guidelines emphasize the primacy of results obtained from history-taking and physical examination, which should then be evaluated in conjunction with the invasiveness and complexity of the surgical procedure. These 2007 guidelines consider ambulatory surgery as one entity, and rate all ambulatory procedures as low risk, with a cardiac mortality <1%. Thus, in the absence of the four active cardiac conditions previously mentioned, additional preoperative interventions or testing would rarely alter the perioperative risk for low-risk procedures such as eye surgery and are not warranted. It cannot be overemphasized, however, that a thorough history and physical examination that can identify the presence or absence of active cardiac conditions is mandatory.

Increasingly, patients with coronary artery disease are undergoing stent placement. A frequently asked question in this context is how long one should wait after stent placement before having elective surgery under general anaesthesia.

Current ACC/AHA Guidelines recommend waiting 4–6 weeks after a bare metal stent, and at least one year after insertion of a drug-eluting stent, until endothelialization is complete. If the patient is at high risk of stent thrombosis, such as those with bifurcated lesions, long stents, diabetes mellitus, renal failure, or a low ejection fraction, dual antiplatelet therapy should be continued for longer than one year. Moreover, elective non-cardiac surgery is not recommended within 4 weeks of coronary revascularization with balloon angioplasty.

Pacemakers and defibrillators

As the demographic profile of contemporary society becomes increasingly geriatric, patients with a cardiac rhythm device (either a pacemaker, an implantable cardiac defibrillator [ICD], or both) presenting for preoperative evaluation have become commonplace. Importantly, the indication for the device must be fully understood, because its presence is often reflective of major underlying cardiac disease.

Permanent pacemakers are typically installed for:

- Symptomatic third-degree heart block
- Type II second-degree heart block

- Sinus node dysfunction
- Recurrent neurally mediated syncope
- Some types of cardiomyopathy

For example, biventricular pacemakers are considered in patients with notable heart failure (ejection fraction <35%) who have not responded sufficiently to medical therapy. ICDs are indicated in patients who sustained a cardiac arrest secondary to a non-temporary problem, including such conditions as:

- Ischaemia
- Long QT syndrome
- Hypertrophic or familial cardiomyopathy

Based on the indication for the device, the patient may not be an appropriate candidate for ophthalmic surgery on an outpatient basis. However, if the patient and procedure are appropriate for the outpatient venue, then basic information about the device should be obtained well in advance of the scheduled surgery to determine whether device interrogation or reprogramming by qualified personnel will be necessary and to allow sufficient time to coordinate the logistical issues.

That said, it should be pointed out that the majority of ophthalmic surgical procedures use minimal bipolar cautery. For some, such as clear-corneal cataract surgery, no cautery is used. Thus, there is a low probability of electromagnetic interference triggering discharge of the device. Indeed, a retrospective survey of ophthalmic anaesthesia providers disclosed that >80% did not use a magnet to reprogramme or inactivate an ICD before surgery.

Further reading

Lee TH, Marcantonio ER, Mangione CM, et al. Derivation and prospective validation of a simple index for prediction of cardiac risk of major noncardiac surgery. *Circulation.* 1999; 100: 1043–9.

Physiologic principles, pharmacologic agents, and techniques of general anaesthesia

Ophthalmic surgery may confer greater hazard than many other types of procedures for laterality errors.

In an attempt to ensure proper patient, operative site, and procedure selection, a tripartite policy involves:

- Preoperative verification of the patient's identity, as well as the proposed nature and site of surgery
- Marking of the intended site
- A 'time-out' immediately before surgery is commenced

It is hoped that adherence to this policy will prevent errors that might otherwise have occurred owing to dysfunctional oral or written communication.

Patients who require or prefer GA for ophthalmic surgery experience a favourable outcome provided:

- The airway is properly maintained
- Haemodynamic stability is achieved
- The globe is kept motionless
- Intra-ocular pressure (IOP) is maintained

The latter is especially important during open-eye operations such as corneal transplantation or open-sky vitrectomy when potential complications such as vitreous loss or expulsive choroidal haemorrhage are feared.

Non-anaesthetic topical agents are increasingly used in the control of IOP. It is imperative to appreciate that drugs given to effect pupillary dilation or to reduce IOP may be absorbed systemically from the conjunctiva or from the nasal mucosa after drainage through the nasolacrimal duct.

- Nasolacrimal duct occlusion is an effective means to minimize systemic absorption, which can have notable anaesthetic implications
- Topical administration of drugs should be avoided in eyes with open conjunctival wounds
- Examples of potentially worrisome topical ocular drugs include cyclopentolate, echothiophate iodide, epinephrine, and timolol

Anaesthesia and intra-ocular agents have important anaesthetic ramifications and are also associated with intra-ocular agents:

- Nitrous oxide, for example, should not be administered concomitantly in patients who receive intra-ocular air or gas
- Nitrous oxide should be discontinued 15–20min before an intravitreous air or gas injection given to tamponade a detached retina
- Discontinuance of nitrous oxide should avoid substantial changes in the volume of the injected bubble and associated changes in IOP
- Furthermore, should the patient require a repeat operation after intravitreous gas injection, the traditional recommendation is to omit nitrous oxide for 5 days after an air injection and for 10 days after a sulphur hexafluoride injection. The nitrous oxide proscription should

be in effect for longer than 30 days if perfluoropropane has been injected (see 📖 General anaesthetic technique, p. 254).

Importantly, resorption time is not always predictable or uniform. There are published cases where a 19-year-old woman with type 1 diabetes injected with sulphur hexafluoride 25 days before subsequent surgery and a 37-year-old male insulin-dependent diabetic injected with perfluoropropane gas 41 days before subsequent surgery were given nitrous oxide and developed central retinal artery occlusion and permanent blindness in the affected eye. Because the pressure in retinal arteries is lower in patients with diabetes, the elderly, and those with atherosclerosis, these patients appear to be at greater risk for this devastating complication.

In some venues, hospital band-type warning bracelets are given to patients who receive intra-ocular gas to alert other clinicians to the presence of the bubble and the need to avoid administration of nitrous oxide.

Anaesthesia field avoidance

Because the anaesthetist is typically positioned remote from the patient's airway, it is mandatory to meticulously secure either the endotracheal tube or the LMA. All connections should be firmly secured because movement of the head by the surgeon might dislodge a weak connection. The contralateral eye should be taped shut and a shield applied to prevent injury. Some ophthalmologists request that the patient's nares be packed with gauze to prevent nasal secretions from contaminating the eye during surgery.

Supraglottic airway versus endotracheal intubation

LMA has gained enormous popularity during the past two decades in patients with minimal risk factors for aspiration. LMA is not only safe and effective for use during eye surgery, but it also offers the advantage of smaller increase in IOP on insertion and removal than is encountered with an endotracheal tube. Having the advantage of being easy to position without laryngoscopy or muscle relaxants, the LMA does not produce the same degree of vasopressor reflexes seen with endotracheal intubation and is less likely to cause dental injury. Vigilance must be maintained to detect initial misplacement or intraoperative displacement of the LMA.

It is essential to appreciate that many geriatric patients have an incompetent oesophagogastric junction and that diabetes is often associated with gastroparesis. These patients, and others with notable risk factors for aspiration, may be managed conservatively by intubation with a cuffed endotracheal tube to protect the lungs. A flexible LMA has a wire reinforced shank that allows it to be repositioned intraoperatively without displacing its seated cuff. It may be useful for oculoplastic procedures that require mucosal grafting. These devices can be more difficult to place. Use of a spatula introducer stiffens the shank and eases placement.

Anaesthetic agents

A wide selection of appropriate anaesthetic agents for ocular surgery is available. Virtually any of the inhalation agents can be administered after intravenous induction with a barbiturate or propofol. Alternatively, a total intravenous anaesthetic technique with a propofol infusion and other intravenous adjuncts can be chosen.

Because it is consistently associated with less postoperative nausea and vomiting than other agents, propofol is an excellent drug for ophthalmic patients.

- Recovery from propofol is rapid and typically associated with a sense of well-being, even euphoria, making it a very suitable drug for ambulatory surgery
- Propofol also attenuates the hypertensive response to intubation and reduces IOP, similar to most intravenous anaesthetic drugs used during eye surgery, such as narcotics and other sedative-hypnotics
- In patients with coronary artery or other types of heart disease, the cardiodepressant effects of propofol can be unwelcome
- Although induction with intravenous etomidate may be more benign in terms of the cardiovascular system, the agent can precipitate postoperative nausea and vomiting and possibly also produce short-term depression of adrenocortical function

If endotracheal intubation is necessary, the selection of the optimal muscle relaxant to facilitate laryngoscopy is made after assessing:

- Patient's airway anatomy
- Probable degree of difficulty of intubation
- Presence or absence of symptomatic reflux
- Haemodynamic consequences of the neuromuscular blocking agent
- Estimated duration of the operation

Although satisfactory control of blood pressure is always important, it has critical implications for retinal perfusion in patients undergoing vitreoretinal surgery.

- If the patient's mean arterial pressure is markedly reduced, retinal perfusion may be inadequate and compromise the visual outcome
- Alternatively, an excessive elevation of retinal arteriole pressure can be dangerous

It therefore behoves the anaesthetist to be cognizant of the patient's usual blood pressure and to strive to maintain haemodynamic parameters within an acceptable range for each individual patient.

A variety of inhalation agents, including isoflurane, desflurane, and sevoflurane, are available for intraoperative maintenance of anaesthesia.

- All these drugs reduce IOP in a dose-dependent fashion, provided oxygenation and ventilation are satisfactorily maintained
- Sevoflurane and, especially, desflurane have lower blood-gas solubilities than all previously used potent inhaled agents
- Theoretically, this solubility advantage should permit greater control of anaesthetic depth and more rapid recovery from general anaesthesia

Regardless of which agent is selected, it should be carefully titrated.

Because akinesia may be indicated for delicate ocular surgery, administration of a non-depolarizing muscle relaxant may be advisable, in conjunction with peripheral nerve monitoring to ensure a twitch height suppression of 90–95%, during open-eye surgery.

Monitoring

Ventilation should be controlled and end-tidal CO_2 continuously monitored to avoid hypercarbia and its ocular hypertensive effect as well as to detect inadvertent disconnection of the endotracheal tube from the anaesthesia circuit, a dangerous event that can be obscured by the surgical drapes. Continuous monitoring of arterial oxygen saturation by pulse oximetry is also essential.

Emergence from anaesthesia

After completion of surgery, any residual neuromuscular block should be reversed. A few minutes before extubation, intravenous lidocaine can be given to prevent or minimize peri-extubation coughing and its deleterious effect on IOP.

- Based on such factors as the patient's airway anatomy, nil per os status, and history of reflux, either awake or deep extubation may be selected
- In experienced hands, either approach is satisfactory for patients who were fasting, who have normal airway anatomy, and who have no risk factors for reflux

Postoperative nausea and vomiting: prevention and therapy

Postoperative nausea and vomiting (PONV) account for a major proportion of unanticipated admissions to hospital after intended ambulatory eye surgery, especially in children (see 📖 Postoperative nausea and vomiting (PONV) p. 218).

PONV is not only distressing to patients; it also has detrimental effects on IOP and can even result in wound dehiscence and admission to an in-patient bed. PONV is more likely to occur after narcotic-based anaesthesia or volatile agents. The incidence is lowest with a total intravenous technique with propofol.

The emetic effects of anaesthetics are modulated in the chemoreceptor trigger zone, where serotonergic, histaminic, muscarinic, and dopaminergic receptors are found. Input also comes from vagal and other stimulation directly to the emetic centre. Although pharmacologic agents that act on the chemoreceptor trigger zone are well represented in our anaesthetic armamentarium, the neurokinin 1 (NK1) antagonists are the only available antiemetics that act on the vomit centre.

Available antiemetics include:
- Benzamides such as metoclopramide
- Butyrophenones such as droperidol
- Phenothiazines such as prochlorperazine
- These three classes of drugs antagonize dopamine receptors
- Scopolamine and atropine are anticholinergics that antagonize muscarinic receptors
- Dimenhydrinate, diphenhydramine, and hydroxyzine antagonize histamine receptors
- Other useful antiemetics include steroids such as dexamethasone and assorted agents such as propofol and ephedrine
- Newer drugs include non-peptide NK1 receptor antagonists and the 5-HT$_3$ serotonergic receptor antagonists, such as ondansetron, tropisetron, ganisetron, and palonosetron

The 5-HT$_3$ blockers are attractive because of the paucity of side effects associated with their use. Unlike many other antiemetics, which can cause drowsiness, dry mouth, or extrapyramidal symptoms, the 5-HT$_3$ antagonists have a relatively clean profile, except for headache and mild effects on liver function. However, like droperidol, some of the drugs in this category can prolong the QT interval. Unlike dropiderol, however, these drugs have not been subject to a black box warning from the Food and Drug Administration. The newest 5-HT$_3$ blocker, palonosetron, has the advantages of a long half-life and no QT-interval issues. And while the 5-HT$_3$ blockers are classically believed to lack efficacy with regard to preventing or treating nausea, palonosetron appears to reduce its severity, and the extended benefits of palonosetron may last up to 3 days. Although the 5-HT$_3$ receptor antagonists have questionable efficacy against centrally induced emesis, non-peptide NK$_1$ receptor antagonists have demonstrated effectiveness against both peripheral and central emetic stimuli in animal models.

- Aprepitant is a highly selective, brain-penetrating NK_1 receptor antagonist with a long half-life of 9–12h and preclinical efficacy against opioid-induced emesis.
- A recent study was the first to investigate the efficacy and side effect profile of oral aprepitant for the prevention of PONV.
- Aprepitant was superior to ondansetron for prevention of vomiting in the first 24 and 48h, but no notable differences were detected between aprepitant and ondansetron for nausea control, use of rescue drugs, or complete response.

During the past two decades, our knowledge concerning the pathophysiology, prevention, and management of PONV has advanced impressively. We now believe, for example, that universal PONV prophylaxis is not cost-effective. Rather, prophylactic treatment should be directed toward those at increased risk for the complication.

Apfel identified a simplified risk score that identified four major risk factors:

- Female gender
- Non-smoking status
- History of PONV
- Opioid use

In his investigation of inpatients receiving balanced inhaled anaesthesia the incidence of PONV with none, one, two, three, or all four risk factors was approximately 10%, 20%, 40%, 60%, and 80%, respectively. Apfel and colleagues claimed that, for inpatients, the type of surgery was not an independent risk factor. It has been reported, however, reported that certain ophthalmic procedures, such as strabismus correction, were associated with an increased risk of PONV.

Guidelines have been developed to provide a comprehensive, evidence-based tool for the management of patients at moderate or high risk for PONV. Double and triple antiemetic combinations (each with a different mechanism of action) are recommended prophylactically for patients at highest risk of PONV. Antiemetic rescue therapy should be given to patients who have an emetic episode postoperatively. If PONV occurs within 6h after surgery, patients should not receive a repeat dose of the prophylactic antiemetic(s). Rather, consider a drug from another class.

Open globe full stomach situations

The patient with a penetrating eye injury and a full stomach is challenging. As in all cases of trauma, it is axiomatic that other injuries must be eliminated before surgically addressing the open-eye injury:

• Skull and orbital fractures
• Intracranial trauma associated with subdural or epidural haematoma formation
• Possibility of thoracic or abdominal injury

The risk of blindness in the injured eye that could result from increased IOP producing extrusion of intra-ocular contents must be balanced against the hazard of aspiration as a result of suboptimal airway management.

Although suxamethonium is typically used as part of a rapid-sequence induction technique for the patient with a full stomach having non-ocular surgery, the use of suxamethonium in ocular trauma was considered by some to be controversial owing to the small, transient (<7min duration) increase in IOP caused by the drug. Many ophthalmic anaesthetists currently believe that suxamethonium, except when contraindicated (malignant hyperthermia susceptibility, for example), is the preferred neuromuscular blocking agent in patients with an open globe and full stomach, recognizing that the use of succinylcholine may decline with the introduction of new and improved drugs. Suxamethonium's rapid, consistent onset allows swift, smooth intubating conditions, and airway protection without coughing or straining. Currently available non-depolarizing agents do not provide such excellent intubating conditions as rapidly or predictably.

Moreover, it is not always possible to foretell which patients may be difficult to intubate or ventilate. The expeditious return of spontaneous respiration is often invaluable in the management of a difficult airway. The use of appropriate intubating doses for rapid-sequence induction with non-depolarizing drugs eliminates this helpful option, although the addition of sugammadex to our armamentarium may nullify, or at least mitigate, this potentially hazardous obstacle.

Patients needing GA whose airway evaluation is favourable may occasionally have a contraindication to the administration of sucinylcholine, such as:

• Malignant hyperthermia susceptibility
• Duchenne muscular dystrophy
• Certain types of myotonia

These patients may be managed using sufficiently large doses of a non-depolarizing neuromuscular blocker to permit accelerated onset of paralysis and adequate intubating conditions. Maintenance could then be accomplished with a total intravenous anaesthetic technique.

When confronted with a patient whose airway anatomy suggests potential difficulties, the anaesthetist should consult with the ophthalmologist concerning the likelihood of saving the injured eye.

In selective instances mentioned previously in which the ocular damage is less serious, the eye is non-salvageable, or the patient with moderate risk factors for GA, GA may be avoided by proceeding under topical or RA. If this approach is not feasible owing to extensive ocular damage (probably rendering the eye non-salvageable), awake fibreoptic laryngoscopy and intubation may be the safest approach, realizing that substantial increases in IOP may occur in conjunction with gagging, retching, and coughing. These risks, however, recede into the background when balanced against the hazard of losing the airway.

Further reading

Conclusion

Although the majority of ophthalmic surgical procedures are performed with RA techniques, GA may be prudent in several circumstances. Because the complications of ophthalmic anaesthesia can be vision-threatening or life-threatening, it is imperative that the anaesthetist appreciates the complex and dynamic interaction among patient diseases, anaesthetic agents, ophthalmic drugs, and surgical manipulation. Effective communication and planning are integral to safe and efficient perioperative care.

Further reading

Apfel CC, Laara E, Koivuranta M, *et al.* A simplified risk score for predicting postoperative nausea and vomiting. *Anesthesiology.* 1999; 91: 693–700.

Fleisher LA, Beckman JA, Brown KA, *et al.* ACC/AHA 2007 Guidelines on perioperative cardiovascular evaluation and care for noncardiac surgery. *Circulation.* 2007; 116: 1971–96.

Gan TJ, Apfel CC, Kovac AL, *et al.* A randomized, double-blind comparison of the NK1 receptor antagonist, aprepitant, versus ondansetron for the prevention of postoperative nausea and vomiting. *Anesth. Analg.* 2007; 104: 1082–9.

Lamb K, James MFM, Janicki PK. The laryngeal mask airway for intraocular surgery: effects on intraocular pressure and stress responses. *Br. J. Anaesth.* 1992; 69: 143–7.

Lee TH, Marcantonio ER, Mangione CM, *et al.* Derivation and prospective validation of a simple index for prediction of cardiac risk of major noncardiac surgery. *Circulation.* 1999; 100: 1043–9.

McGoldrick KE. Ocular pathology and systemic diseases: anesthetic implications. In KE McGoldrick, ed., *Anesthesia for ophthalmic and otolaryngologic surgery.* Philadelphia: WB Saunders; 1992: 210–26.

McGoldrick KE. What is the best technique in the patient with an open globe and full stomach? In LA Fleisher ed., *Evidence-based practice of anesthesia.* Philadelphia: Elsevier; 2009: 2926–99.

Schein OD, Katz J, Bass EB, *et al.* The value of routine preoperative medical testing medical testing before cataract surgery. *N. Engl. J. Med.* 2000; 342: 168–75.

Scott IU, McCabe CM, Flynn Jr HW, *et al.* Local anesthesia with intravenous sedation for surgical repair of selected open-globe injuries. *Am. J. Ophthalmol.* 2002; 134: 707–11.

Seaberg RR, Freeman WR, Goldbaum MH, Manecke GR. Permanent postoperative vision loss associated with expansion of intraocular gas in the presence of a nitrous oxide-containing anesthetic. *Anesthesiology.* 2002; 97: 1309–10.

Stoller GL. Ophthalmic surgery and the implantable cardioverter defibrillator. *Arch. Ophthalmol.* 2006; 124: 123–5.

Tattersall FD, Rycroft W, Francis B, *et al.* Tachykinin NK1 receptor antagonists act centrally to inhibit emesis induced by the chemotherapeutic agent cisplatin in ferrets. *Neuropharmacology.* 1996; 35: 1121–9.

Zaidan JR, Atlee JL, Belott P, *et al.* for the American Society of Anesthesiologists task force on perioperative management of patients with cardiac rhythm management devices. Practice advisory for the perioperative management of patients with cardiac rhythm devices: pacemakers and implantable cardioverter-defibrillators. *Anesthesiology.* 2005; 103: 186–98.

Chapter 12

Anaesthetic considerations in the elderly

Professor Chris Dodds

Introduction

Over the next couple of decades the demands made by an increasingly elderly population will challenge all healthcare systems across the globe. Whilst there are many simple ophthalmic surgical procedures that can be safely performed under regional orbital blockade there are those that will continue to require the safe provision of GA. Some aspects of this will be covered in this chapter.

Background

The age distribution of the populations across the world has been changing rapidly with a fall in birth rate leading to lower numbers of people entering employment at the same time that death rates have fallen because of improved public health services, pharmaceutical innovations, and therapeutic developments. This has adversely altered the 'dependency ratio' (the number of workers against the number being supported by them) leading to a growing inability for a nationally based health service to pay for all care needed by their populations.

- This is going to get worse until approximately 2050 after which the 'baby-boomers' will have moved on!
- This imbalance between supporting and supported sections of society is also influenced by the progressive changes due to ageing and chronic disease. Loss of independence of an individual requires (usually) another family member to provide care for them
- As a population ages the carer may themselves be infirm and it will not be at all uncommon for a 70-year-old to be looking after a frail 90-year-old parent. Clearly the burden is likely to fall onto the 45-year-old sibling who is not only having to work but also support their own children through higher education. This domino sequence will fail if any of these links breaks down

There are many currently untreatable causes of dependency that increase with advancing age such as dementia and stroke, but visual impairment is both common and often treatable. The commonest by far is cataract, followed by glaucoma and then age-related macular degeneration, and treating these will often reverse dependency in all societies.

Whilst the treatment and anaesthesia for these conditions is covered elsewhere in this book, the underlying changes with ageing have to be clearly understood and embedded into anaesthesia and surgical practice.

Changes in the elderly

Changes in the elderly

The underlying cellular changes that occur as longevity develops are being elucidated and there is clear variation in when these occur across population groups. The various theories as to why we age range from programmed death, accumulation of toxic metabolites, or failure of immune processes to the failure of effective genetic replication. Whatever the processes, there are some markers of ageing we can identify. These may be best understood by consideration of the changes that occur within cellular systems, within organs, and within integrated systems. The overarching behavioural responses to these changes should not be underestimated as this is the 'visible' response we can observe in aging patients.

Cellular changes

Continuous cellular repair and regeneration is essential to maintain organ and organism health.

- The various processes include activation and specialization of progenitor/stem cells to replace damaged cells to the sequestration of metabolic fragments of intracellular proteins. Intracellular processes may also trigger cell death (apoptosis) as part of a programmed response to irretrievable damage. The breadth and detail of these is beyond this review but some examples include the following.

- Progenitor (stem) cell function declines with age despite the remaining presence of these cells in the majority of organ systems. There appears to be a blocking of the 'notch' receptors that trigger differentiation of the stem cells into their final morphological state. Research in rodents has demonstrated a reversal of this apparent inactivation in muscle progenitor cells by transfusing blood from younger animals with a subsequent restoration of stem cell activation. This suggestion of a humoural factor inhibiting stem cell function has interesting therapeutic implications for us. There is also an apparent sex difference as females maintain telomere length on replication more than males, as seen in myocyte regeneration.

- The metabolic processes that lead ultimately to an intracellular accumulation of β-amyloid, the recognized cellular defect in dementia, can be genetically modified (at least in mice). Modification of the genetic sequencing, to cause either enhancement of the metabolism of protein breakdown products that lead to β-amyloid production or suppression, prevented onset of dementia-like signs in susceptible mice when the effector gene was switched off.

- Interest in the role of the astrocyte within the central nervous system has grown as it is now identified as a major influence in neuronal responses to injury. Once thought of as no more than a form of skeletal support for the axonal cells, it is now recognized as a complex syncitium capable of responding to injury and mounting a response that may last for years if not decades. Common insults such as ischaemia, haemorrhage, anaesthesia or head injury may trigger an increase in inducible nitric oxide synthetase (iNOS), an increase in apoptosis, a synergistic response with apolipoprotein ε-4 and also production of heat shock proteins. Once the astrocytes have been activated by

trauma they remain responsive to even minor degrees of injury such as transient hypoxia for many months if not years. Such activation may provide an insight into the unpredictable onset of postoperative cognitive dysfunction.
- One of the most robust intracellular control systems is that for electrolyte balance. This is tightly maintained throughout life with little change in the electrical membrane potentials or serum and cellular ion concentrations. If there is a marked imbalance, hyponatraemia for example, without an identifiable cause such as renal failure, this has to be recognized as a very significant and potentially end-of-life dysfunction.

Organ changes

Functional reserve for the majority of organs systems decreases with age. This follows both structural changes and alterations in homeostatic mechanisms:
- An example of where structural changes affect function can be seen in the kidneys, where a loss of cortical nephrons leads to a reduction in the osmotic gradient across the counter-current system and a fall in the kidney's ability to alter rapidly the concentration of urine and also limiting the extent of such homeostasis. Homeostatic deterioration is often seen in the orthostatic baroreceptor responses. Sudden changes in posture, such as sitting up from the recumbent position, may lead to profound hypotension and fainting. This autonomic dysfunction occurs despite the circulating levels of catecholamines being several times higher than in young subjects. There is a sympathetic downregulation and responsiveness to postural changes relies on inhibition of the vagal parasympathetic tone.
- It is this change in autonomic performance that explains to poor response in the elderly to indirect sympathomimetics such as ephedrine.

Systematic changes

Other anaesthetically important changes may involve deterioration in a combination of systems.
- An example is the gradual reduction in the sensitivity of the cough reflex with age. By the age of 70 this is approximately 7 times less sensitive to potent airway irritants.
- The concurrent fall in tone of the gastrooesophageal sphincter and partial upper airway obstruction make oesophageal reflux a frequent occurrence. Recurrent asymptomatic aspiration is common in the over 80 population. This has clear implications to the use of supraglottic airway devices.
- The reduced sensitivity to airway stimulation also leads to an attenuation of the response to intubation. The use of local anaesthetic sprays directly onto the vocal cords can lead to significant systemic absorption and cause hypotension.
- Complex processing within the central nervous system, especially those areas that maintain vigilance or cognition, are more vulnerable with advancing age. There is less cell loss than originally thought with age but certainly cell size is reduced and synaptic connections

may be attenuated. The incidence of inattention and frank dementia increases independently with age. Progressive failure of the adrenergic and cholinergic systems respectively are believed to underlie these conditions.

- What is clear is that there is a subclinical deterioration long before signs are apparent in both of these states and also that once evident the decline in function affects many other systems.
- Dementia, for example, affects not only memory and cognition but also gastrointestinal function and motor function. Even if patients are identified as having mild cognitive impairment this does not predict cognitive dysfunction following surgery.

Behavioural adaptation

In common with many mammals humans will adapt their behaviour in response to limited function. This is seen across the organ systems in the elderly including the CNS, locomotor, renal, and gastrointestinal systems.

- Early dementia or mild cognitive dysfunction is more common than usually anticipated and adaption may present simply as a loss of confidence in an individual, in their increasing reliance on notes or carers attending consultations with them. Loss of the behavioural response to hypothermia is present in about 20% of the elderly and follows a blunting of their hypothalamic thermostatic control.
- It is also important to identify the interplay between their medical care and an individual's dignity and self-esteem. Oral fluid intake will be actively restricted if there is an incontinence problem or uncertainty in being able to actually get to the toilet due to arthritis or after trauma, no matter how determined their carers' are.

Pain management

Both acute and chronic pain is poorly managed in the elderly.

- This is partly due to a lack of appropriate pain-scoring systems specifically for the elderly and also due to a reluctance to prescribe effective analgesics.
- There is no evidence at all that the elderly do not feel pain to the same degree as younger patients, although their means of expressing it may well differ. Vocabulary is dynamic and the very words used by the elderly to describe 'absolute agony' may be 'painful'.

Discussion of the impact of chronic pain is beyond the remit of this chapter, but management of acute postoperative pain in the ophthalmic patient should be just as vigorous as in younger patients.

- Recording pain scores and identifying what action has been taken are essential requirements in patient care in the UK (the 5th vital sign) and recommended internationally.
- There should be no hesitation in prescribing effective doses of opiates if required, although dose titration may be needed.

General anaesthetic aspects

Consent

Capacity fluctuates and must be assessed formally whenever consent is sought or changes to a procedure planned.

- The legal status of informed consent varies across the world but the principles underlying it are constant.
- The expected standard is that all attempts will be made, using appropriate methods of communication, to ensure that the patient understands the implications of the procedure and its outcome.
- Even during a routine preoperative assessment patients (of all ages) do not understand up to 45% of the technical terms used by doctors. An example would be where an infective cause for a degree of delirium is identified and the surgery is not of an immediate nature. In this situation consent should wait until the infection has been effectively treated and cognitive function confirmed as having returned to their normal level.
- Where there is an identified dysfunction it is wise to seek a formal psychogeriatric opinion before proceeding further.

Assessment

Elderly patient's conditions change rapidly because of the limitation of functional reserve and a variable response to infective or biochemical challenges.

- Whilst pre-assessment systems are becoming routine the recorded findings need to be reviewed on the day of admission for any change to the ASA status since primary review.
- An evaluation of medication actually being taken is necessary, those that have been prescribed as well as any proprietary ones: the elderly are prone to stop essential medication if they become unwell because they often blame their symptoms on a prescribed drug.
- If the procedure involves any change in position of the patient's head or neck then awake assessment of their ability to maintain this position without pain or neurological symptoms such as vertigo should be performed and documented. This is especially important if there is a history of medium vessel atherosclerosis.
- Special senses—hearing as well as sight—should be assessed and documented in the postoperative plan as well as preoperatively. Hearing aids with functioning batteries can transform a frightened patient into a relaxed one.

Monitoring

- This should start on the ward or reception area with temperature measurement as well as the more routine cardiovascular variables; heart rate, blood pressure, and oxygen saturation.
- If there is any degree of hypothermia warming should start immediately, with forced air systems where available. It is unacceptable to start ophthalmic surgery in a hypothermic patient.
- Accuracy of the pulse oximeter should be confirmed by comparison of the recorded heart rate with that of the ECG. Any variation, especially

in the presence of atrial fibrillation, should lead to a questioning of the true arterial oxygen saturation.
- Where adhesive pads, for the ECG or electromyograph (EMG) for instance, are used they must balance adhesion with limited damage to the elderly friable thin skin.

Induction

Whether GA or regional techniques are planned venous access has to be considered.
- The onset of LA agents is slightly slower in the elderly but the duration of action may be doubled or more, especially so with the longer-acting agents such as ropivacaine.
- Lipid rescue facilities should be available in all theatres where LA is practiced although there are to date no reports of its use in the elderly.
- For GA in the elderly induction should follow effective pre-oxygenation. Three minutes is not long enough because of their restricted vital capacity and functional reserve especially when supine.
- Estimation of their circulation time is valuable (easily observed if glycophyrrolate is administered IV as a vagolytic and the time to a pulse rate change noted).
- The commonest untoward incident on induction is inadvertent overdose of the induction agent because a lack of loss of verbal responses is attributed to insufficient induction agent rather than patiently waiting for the bolus to reach the patient's brain. Profound hypotension follows with unpredictable neurocognitive and cardiovascular sequelae.
- A similar response time is present when using non-depolarizing neuro-muscular blocking agents. Elderly muscles are no longer vessel-rich as fatty infiltration replaces damaged myocytes. This greatly delays maximal onset of blockade and also delays recovery even after use of reversal agents. The elderly are rarely intubated during full relaxation as this can take up to 9min to occur, but is it common to administer second doses before the first has worked if a nerve stimulator is used after intubation.
- The use of LA sprays to the larynx to modify the cardiovascular response to laryngoscopy has to be viewed with caution as tracheal and pulmonary absorption may lead to direct cardiovascular effects. The dose to be administered should be calculated as if the drug were to be injected intravenously.
- Supraglottic airway devices are used increasingly with success for ophthalmic procedures. The cautions on positioning of the head remain as with intubation. Flexible devices are more appropriate when more access to the face is needed than simple globe-related procedures.
- Airway protection from blood and debris is necessary during naso-lacrimal surgery and the choice of formal intubation or the use of a supraglottic airway may be difficult.
- Patient safety is the paramount consideration but that will be balanced by the knowledge of the surgical team and the experience of the anaesthetist.

Positioning

As mentioned above the elderly have to be assumed to have an unstable cervical spine and treated with extreme care when flexing and extending their head.

- The combination of ligamental laxity and cervical spondylosis make compromise of the cervical cord or compression of the vertebral arteries more likely with advancing age.
- All joints are less mobile and often have a relatively fixed range of movement. Joint surfaces may be arthritic and movement under anaesthesia can cause an arthritic flare in these joints which may be far more painful than the operative pain.
- Use of Trendelenberg positions directly causes changes in IOP, choroidal and optic nerve thickness. These may all be exacerbated during surgery and anaesthesia.
- Pressure from supports is easily identified, but prolonged, more than an hour, procedures run a risk of pressure damage to sacral, scapular, and cephalic skin.
- Standard operating table mattresses may not be adequate protection and gel pads or similar devices should be used.

Maintenance

- The elderly benefit from the use of anaesthetic agents that are either rapidly metabolized to inactive products or volatile agents with minimal lipid solubility. The longer the procedure the more important the context sensitive half-time becomes.
- The use of nitrous oxide is controversial with antagonists believing that there is no place for this agent in modern anaesthesia because of its role in postoperative nausea and vomiting, the risks of hypoxia, the loss of nitrogen splinting of alveoli and the haematological consequences of prolonged use.
- The advantage of a more rapid uptake of volatile anaesthetic agents has become largely academic with the latest generation of agents; sevoflurane and desflurane.
- Xenon is being investigated as an anaesthetic with similar potency to nitrous oxide (and therefore risks of hypoxia) but it is showing promising signs of neuro-protection which may make it clearly indicated in the elderly.
- Indications for hypotension during ophthalmic surgery in the elderly are very limited and demand sophisticated cerebral as well as full invasive cardiovascular monitoring.
- The need for complete paralysis still remains although less frequently than before. It must be assessed and recorded continuously by appropriate monitors such as EMG or 'train of four' devices. Non-steroid relaxants are preferable as they are largely independent of hepatic and renal function.

Recovery

Active recovery management is necessary to ensure the elderly maintain their ventilation, oxygenation, and cardiovascular stability.

- They should be elevated to an semi-sitting position if at all possible before extubation or removal of supraglottic devices.
- Providing their glasses and/or hearing aids before emergence is more likely to avoid disorientation and confusion, as are brightly lit surroundings and the sitting-up position.
- Hypothermia should have been avoided by aggressive management throughout, but if it is identified it should been treated urgently as the oxygen demand from shivering can be hazardous for an elderly patient with poor respiratory or cardiovascular function.
- Airway tone is reduced with age and snoring (partial airway obstruction) seen as an indication for supportive measures. Aspiration is more likely to occur and also less likely to trigger coughing or laryngospasm.
- Thresholds for blood transfusion have to be modified in the elderly, especially if they have limited cardiorespiratory reserve. The 30% drop in haemoglobin to 7GdL that demands a 30% increase in cardiac output for maintenance of oxygen delivery may be just too much to ask for the sake of protocols derived in fitter younger patients.

Conclusion

The skills, knowledge and behaviours required of anaesthetists caring for the elderly exceed those for all other subspecialties. The highly individualized nature of this population rules out all protocol-based management and instead demands that each patient has to be personally assessed, managed, and supported by experienced medical staff. The surgical procedure may be similar but the patient will not be.

As we all benefit from longer (and hopefully) fitter lives, as expectations (including ours) increase much of the ophthalmic healthcare provision will be delivered to those over 65 years of age.

As the subspecialty that underpins all aspects of ophthalmic practice, apart from paediatrics, a thorough understanding of ageing, chronic disease and complex pharmacological cocktails is essential.

Key reading

Babitu U.Q and Cyna A M. Patients' understanding of technical terms used during the pre-anaesthetic consultation. *Anaesth. Intensive Care*. 2010; 38(2): 349–53.

Bekker A, Lee C, Santi S. *et al.* Does mild cognitive impairment increase the risk of developing postoperative cognitive dysfunction? *Am. J. Surg.* 2010; 199(6): 782–8.

Conboy M, Conboy MJ, Wagers AJ, *et al.* Rejuvenation of aged progenitor cells by exposure to a young systemic environment. *Nature*. 2005; 433(7027): 760–4.

Grant GP, Szirth BC, Bennett HL, *et al.* Effects of prone and reverse Trendelenburg positioning on ocular parameters. *Anesthesiology*. 2010; 112(1): 57–65.

Kajstura J, Gurusamy N, Ogorek B, *et al.* Myocyte turnover in the aging human heart. *Circ. Res.* 2010; 107(11): 1374–86.

Kang H, Park HJ, Baek SK, *et al.* Effects of preoxygenation with the three minutes tidal volume breathing technique in the elderly. *Korean J. Anesthesiol*. 2010; 58(4): 369–73.

Li M, Bertout JA, Ratcliffe SJ, *et al.* Acute anemia elicits cognitive dysfunction and evidence of cerebral cellular hypoxia in older rats with systemic hypertension. *Anesthesiology*. 2010; 113(4): 845–58.

Lockwood G. Theoretical context-sensitive elimination times for inhalation anaesthetics. *Br. J. Anaesth*. 2010; 104(5): 648–55.

Ma D, Wilhelm S, Maze M, *et al.* Neuroprotective and neurotoxic properties of the 'inert' gas, xenon. *Br. J. Anaesth*. 2002; 89(5): 739–46.

Paqueron X, Boccara G, Bendahou M, *et al.* Brachial plexus nerve block exhibits prolonged duration in the elderly. *Anesthesiology*. 2002; 97(5): 1245–9.

Shu Y, Patel S M, Pac-Soo C, *et al.* Xenon pretreatment attenuates anesthetic-induced apoptosis in the developing brain in comparison with nitrous oxide and hypoxia. *Anesthesiology*. 2010; 113(2): 360–8.

Sieber FE (Ed.) *Geriatric anesthesia*. New York: McGraw-Hill; 2007.

Uchinda L, Sukchareon I, Kusumaphanyo C, *et al.* The Thai Anesthesia Incident Monitoring Study (Thai AIMS): an analysis of perioperative complication in geriatric patients. *J. Med. Assoc. Thai.* 2010; 93(6): 698–707.

Chapter 13

Anaesthesia for paediatric ophthalmic surgery

Dr Jacqueine Tutiven

Introduction

At birth, the eye measures close to three-quarters that of the adult eye, reaching adult size by 14 years of age. The posterior portion grows proportionately more than the anterior portion of the globe. Infants do not see as well as adults. Infant's psychophysical sensitivity to light, colour, and contrast are far below the comparable values in adults, especially between 1 and 4 months. Infant visual acuity is poor at birth. At birth, visual acuity (VA) is approximately 20/400 to 20/800. By 4 to 5 months infants are no longer 'legally blind' (e.g., 20/200). VA reaches 20/20 between 8 to 12 months and does not reach the adult value until at least 3 years. Visual acuity can not be measured accurately until the age of 3 months. The infant's sclera is thin, translucent, and bluish in colour. The cornea measures 10mm and the curvature of the eye eventually flattens out with growth. The newborn has a fully developed retina but the fovea is immature.

Newborns can immediately explore their surroundings, whether in total darkness or upon a lit environment. Their eye movements depend on exogenous and endogenous control not necessarily dependent on visual sensory feedback signals. Eye movement in the dark reflects endogenous control; they are frequent and controlled. Extrinsic control of eye movements depends on the visual sensorial stimulation. Newborns can methodically scan high-contrast contour areas.

Preoperative assessment

During the preoperative visit, a brief discussion with the parents and or caregiver should be undertaken to review the perinatal history and to go over any hospital discharge medical records pertinent to the patient's current status. This is especially true for infants held in the neonatal unit for an extended period of time after birth. Important factors to consider are:

- Neonatal history
- Conceptual age
- Surgery
- Medication history
- Review of past anaesthetics

A brief summary of the mother's pregnancy, her medical issues and/or any issues that may have contributed to a tumultuous birth with possible anoxic injury to the infant should be questioned since it may relate with poor autoregulatory response of the cerebral circulation due to vasoparalysis.

Although most paediatric patients are healthy, some infants and children that present for ophthalmic examinations and surgery may have concomitant systemic disorders or syndromes that will need to be addressed during the preoperative visit. In these cases one should inquire about:

- Metabolic deficiencies
- Neuromuscular disorders
- Muscular dystrophies
- Cardiorespiratory issues

Apnoea of prematurity

Sleep disorders

With common syndromes that accompany ophthalmopathies, dysmorphic features of the head and face make it imperative to address airway issues and obstructive sleep disorders.

Any prolonged stay in a neonatal unit after birth or during infancy may suggest treatment needed to have helped the baby transition to a viable neonatal state. Most premature babies do well with supportive care and within controlled environments to allow them to thrive outside of the Neonatal Intensive Care Unit (NICU) within a short time. Because the gestational age limit of viability has declined to a point where in some units 50% of neonates born at 24 weeks gestation may survive, these extreme premature babies do so only after going through extensive neonatal respiratory and circulatory support, surgical interventions, and other life-sustaining treatments.

Factors that play a role in the risk of having apnoea of prematurity are:

- A post-conceptual age less than 60 weeks with supportive respiratory treatments and/or medications with apnoea monitoring
- Anaemia
- Developmental immaturity: low gestational age and brainstem immaturity sets the scene for central clinical apnoea due to immature brainstem neuronal function

- **Neuromodulators**: both excitatory and inhibitory neuromodulators for respiration are imbalanced in the premature infant promoting an unstable respiratory pattern in newborn infants
- **Altered sleep state**: this instability of respiratory control is widely appreciated during the rapid eye movements (REM) cycle of sleep in the premature neonate and may be influenced by cortical factors
- **Chemoreceptor responses**: premature infants do not respond to increases in carbon dioxide levels, unlike normal term or older infants. Hypoxia is also met with a different response from the preterm neonate. Here, a transient hyperventilation is soon followed by hypoventilation and apnoea. This is not to be confused with physiologic periodic breathing seen and measured commonly in newborns
- **Respiratory muscles coordination**: the immature and/or depressed respiratory drive to the muscles of respiration, together with a reduction in electromyographic activity seen in the diaphragm of premature and syndromic babies during spontaneous obstructive breathing are key factors that explain central and obstructive apnoea. Apnoeic spells and irregular breathing is compounded with the relative relaxation of skeletal muscle tone, which in turn worsens lung expansion during inspiration due to the highly compliant chest wall
- **Depressed laryngeal reflexes**: muscles of the upper airway, especially the genioglossus, have shown a delay in response to the hypercapnoea in comparison with the diaphragm, for as much as one minute. Along with a compliant pharynx that may collapse under negative inspiratory pressures, gastrooesophageal reflux (GOR) also plays a role by exciting chemoreceptors in the larynx that signal the medulla to elicit apnoea

Physical examination

There are age-related differences in the physical examination findings.
- The child's overall ability to thrive reflects a state of well-being
- A generalized assessment of the infant's growth, weight and cardiorespiratory rates may provide an initial global appreciation of the child's status

Airway considerations

A child may be predisposed to perioperative airway obstruction because of the differences seen in the function, oro-pharyngeal dimensions and the presence of hypertrophic tonsils, dysmorphic features, and presence of an upper respiratory infection.
- Large occiput gives neonates and infants a natural 'sniffing position' assisting in aligning their airway for patency. A small roll may be placed under their shoulders to improve laryngoscopic view
- Small mouth aperture and a large tongue in relation to the size of the mouth may obstruct laryngoscopic view
- Mandible is small and the neck is short
- The larynx lies at the level of C3–4
- The larynx antero-cephalad with a stiff short epiglottis
- In children between the ages of 6 and 8, one must examine for loose teeth

Cardiovascular considerations

- Colour at rest and while crying, perfusion state, palpable pulses
- The cardiac heart sounds in the newborn—S1 and S2, murmurs or clicks may be present
- Heart rate increases in the first two months of life then stabilizes gradually in childhood
- The neonatal heart has limited cardiac reserve
- Beta stimulation at birth and effects of thyroid hormones explains the newborn's increased cardiac contractility
- An infant's resting heart operates at a higher preload, afterload, contractility and heart rate
- Heart rate plays the most important factor in cardiac function
- Acceptable heart rates are:
  - Infants 100–180 beats per minute (bpm)
  - Infants to toddlers 80–150bpm
  - >Than 3 years to 10 years old 70–110bpm
- Syndromic children with arrhythmias may have:
  - Congenital cardiac diseases
  - First-, second-, or third-degree heart blocks
  - Supraventricular tachycardias (SVTs)
- Features that increase the risk of presenting a cardiac pathology include:
  - Malformation syndromes
  - Increased precordial activity
  - Abnormal heart sounds (clicks and loud or harsh murmurs)
  - Decreased femoral pulses

A preoperative anaesthesia evaluation of the child with a significant cardiac dysfunction should include:

- An updated comprehensive paediatric cardiology evaluation for surgery
- Electrocardiogram, echocardiography reports
- Haematocrit and haemoglobin level
- Baseline oxygen saturation level on room air
- Chest radiograph and a clear explanation of the type of the cardiac lesion

Nervous system considerations

Factors to take note of during the history and exam for the neuromuscular system are:

- Head trauma
- Hydrocephalus
- History of or existence of CNS tumours
- Developmental delay
- Motor dysfunction
- Neuromuscular diseases and muscle diseases
- There is reduced predictability of the pharmacokinetics of the anaesthetic drugs, narcotics, and adjuvants in neuromuscular compromised children than healthy children
- Suxamethonium may be contraindicated in children with muscular diseases, myotonias or generalized hypotonia

- Many researchers have proven a direct relation of metabolic hyperthermic reactions and malignant hyperthermia to inhalation agents and suxamethonium in children with muscular disorders, especially Duchenne's muscular dystrophy

Gastrointestinal considerations

- Gastrooesophageal reflux may present in normal infants. Risk of aspiration and increased oral secretions are greater and commonly seen in these children
- If parents give a history of repeated respiratory infections, wheezing, or bronchial infections, there may be an increased chance of perioperative aspiration and the infant or child should be considered 'at risk'

Separation anxiety and premedication

Separation anxiety is a well-described concern of paediatric patients and their families. The preoperative visit and the presence of parents during induction of general anaesthesia relieve anxiety in many children. Still, others may undergo preoperative stress and parents find relief offering their children a mild sedative to decrease their stress.

- All children receiving anxiolytics and sedatives should be appropriately monitored and hospital paediatric sedation policies should be followed
- Anxiolytics can be administered intramuscularly, intranasally, by mouth, by rectum or intravenously

Oral midazolam

Oral midazolam (0.5mg/kg; maximum 20mg) is a formidable pre-surgical anxiolytic although its pharmacokinetic profile may make its effect less predictable.

- Onset of effect is 10–15min
- Duration approximately 60min
- Midazolam, when given in standard doses, will not prolong emergence or discharge from the hospital
- Nasal midazolam (0.2mg/kg)
- May induce burning sensation in the mucosa and crying

Oral clonidine (2 to 4 mcg/kg)

- Provides anxiolysis within 20–30min
- Decreases the incidence of postoperative nausea and vomiting

Ketamine

A phenylcyclidine derivative, causes anaesthesia and analgesia through its dissociative effects between the thalamus and the limbic cortex, thus temporarily impairing sensory impulses.

- Ketamine increases the heart rate, crosses the blood–brain barrier and increases cerebral blood flow, increases blood pressure, and dilates the bronchial airways
- Spontaneous respiration and pharyngeal–laryngeal reflexes are preserved
- The potential risk for aspiration with ketamine is minimal, but there have been reports of dose-related airway reflex impairment seen
- Children have better pharyngeal–laryngeal reflexes with ketamine.

- Ketamine is contraindicated in ill neonates because of an increased incidence of ketamine associated aspiration seen in this group Recommended optimum dose:
- Analgesia: 0.25–0.75mg/kg or 2–4mg/kg IM
- Clinical dissociation: 1–2mg/kg IV or 6–13mg/kg IM. IV doses should be administered over 1min and continuous infusion of ketamine is not recommended in children
- In mentally challenged, attention deficit hyperactivity disorder (ADHD) and autistic children it provides quick predictable onset with relative slow recovery for paediatric sedation together with a wide margin of safety
- Placement of IV lines in combative children: 2.5mg/kg–5mg/kg IM or 1.5–2mg/kg IV
- May be given with midazolam in which case we recommend decreasing the ketamine dose by half
- Ketamine may prolong recovery time and hospital discharge
- Anticipate recovery period from 1–2h. These children usually recover slowly and are less agitated under quiet conditions
- Consider anticholinergic agent because it decreases vagal autonomic stimulation and decreases excessive salivation
- Atropine (0.02mg/kg IM or IV) may cause flushing, dry mouth, hyperthermia and CNS irritability
- Glycopyrrolate (0.01mg/kg IM or IV) minimal CNS effects, less tachycardia

Ophthalmic medications in children

Cycloplegics and mydriatic medications are commonly used preoperatively as part of medical treatment or to prepare the eye for fundoscopy and surgery. Systemic absorption is possible once the solutions enters the lacrimal systems and is absorbed via the nasopharyngeal mucosa.

- Cyclopentolate is a cycloplegic agent that inhibits muscarinic receptors at the ciliary body and inhibits pupillary accommodation secondary to paralysis of the ciliary muscles:
  - Onset of action is 20–40min and its effects may last 36h
  - Side effects include GI discomfort, vomiting, ileus and signs and symptoms of anti-cholinergic toxicity
- Ophthalmic phenylephrine:
  - Available in 2.5% (1.25mg in one drop) and 10% concentrations
  - Achieves pupillary dilation and vasoconstriction within minutes of placement. Usual dosage is one drop of 2.5% per hour
  - Iatrogenic malignant hypertension has been reported therefore full strength 10% phenylephrine should be avoided

Fasting in children

Despite a lack of consensus for optimal fasting intervals for formula-fed infants among paediatric anaesthetists, and the evidence-based clinical studies suggesting gastric fluid volumes at less than what is considered a risk for pulmonary aspiration after a critical time interval, the following fasting recommendations at author's institution are as follows:

- Clear fluids should be allowed 2–3h prior to surgery
- Breast milk is recommended 4h prior to surgery
- Formula is allowed between 4–6h prior to surgery

In practice, avoiding prolonged nil by mouth (NPO) periods decrease the following risks of hypovolaemia, hypoglycaemia and perioperative hypotension.

Retinopathy of prematurity/retinal detachments in infants

The premature retina presents vasoproliferative changes that are categorized in stages I to V. Screening for retinopathy of prematurity (ROP) is commonly performed in the neonatal intensive care units with topical anaesthetic eye drops. Progression of disease may require laser treatments and thus anaesthetic coverage.

Laser treatment and neonatal anaesthesia in the NICU

The ophthalmologist requires a quiet field and a still baby to provide a good examination and successful treatment for threshold ROP with laser in the NICU. Methods and availability for different forms of anaesthesia/analgesia for the laser treatment of ROP in the NICU vary widely. Unless the patient is intubated, on ventilatory support and sedated, the minimum optimal environment can be achieved with:

- Providing external heat and swaddled (wrapped), baby in the supine position and head immobilized
- Pupillary dilatation may be achieved with phenylephrine 2.5% and tropicamide 0.5% as a cycloplegic. A mean pupillary change of up to 0.9mm can be seen, but it is recommended to use cycloplegic agent alone due to these infants' high risk of a rise in blood pressure
- Cyclomydril, a combination of phenylephrine 1% with cyclopentolate 0.2%, delivers lower concentrations with lower incidences of blood pressure changes
- Topical anaesthetic drops, proparacaine hydrochloride 0.5% (Alcaine®) lasts 15min and lidocaine 2% gel may provide a longer duration of safe and effective analgesia without toxicity to ocular surface
- Acetaminophen 30–40mg/kg per rectal (PR) helps
- Sedation/analgesia with fentanyl 0.5–1mg/kg and midazolam 0.05–0.2mg/kg/dose IV. Watch for myoclonus, bradycardia, respiratory depression, and hypotension
- Cardiorespiratory monitoring is essential
- Assisted ventilation appears to be more effective than passive ventilation, over a short period of time, during a procedure in the NICU or within a surgical suite

If a surgical suite is requested for evaluations under anaesthesia (EUA) and laser treatment the following plans may help:

- Mask spontaneous ventilation with a balanced anaesthetic technique.
- LMA with spontaneous ventilation/pressure support ventilation and balanced anaesthetic technique
- Endotracheal anaesthesia with spontaneous ventilation/pressure support ventilation with a balanced anaesthetic technique

Ophthalmic evaluations under anaesthesia in premature children

Ophthalmologic EUAs are undertaken for photography, ultrasound, and visualization of intra-ocular tumours, laser, retinal disease, IOP measurements, and intra-ocular injection of chemotherapy.

- Most infants and children for short EUAs can be safely anaesthetized via facemask GA and allowed to breathe spontaneously
- More comprehensive EUAs with surgery will require IV placement and airway management; anaesthesia is maintained with volatiles in oxygen and nitrous oxide

Ex-premature infants may be recovering from long-term neonatal treatments. For the most part, ventilatory support for hyaline membrane disease in the neonatal units reflects moderately high transpulmonary pressures, with rapid cycles per minute that may at times average around 55 per minute. Despite respiratory tissues healing and developing normally after discharge from neonatal units, these infants might benefit from assisted ventilator settings when undergoing general endotracheal anaesthesia for surgical procedures.

Anaesthetic technique

- Inhalation induction with sevoflurane in O_2 and air. Neonates and premature infants have lower anaesthetic requirements, the minimum alveolar concentration (MAC) value decreases by 20–30%
- IV access for hydration and drug administration
- Dextrose 5% Ringer's lactate
- Glycopyrrolate 0.01–0.02mg/kg IV
- Muscle relaxation is not required for evaluations but if there is a need to provide muscle relaxation and/or the use of a muscle relaxant for intubation, cisatracurium 0.15–0.2mg/kg or atracurium 0.4–0.6mg/kg has advantages in the neonate and infant because of its metabolism
- Adjuvants: propofol (1mg/kg IV) may be given as an adjunct for airway management with an LMA. The addition of a short acting narcotic bolus may also provide for a smooth intubation
- Mask ventilation/LMA/ETT: airway management during these cases is chosen depending on the complexity of the evaluation under general anaesthesia and clinical judgement
- Maintenance: inhalation agents in O_2 and air or N_2O is provided with an O_2 saturation between 90–95% that should reflect PaO^2 levels between 60–80mmHg
- Modes of ventilation: if the procedure is short and the neonates' condition is healthy, spontaneous ventilation is acceptable. Pressure support modes are favourable when the patient has an LMA or ETT
- Emergence: patients are usually allowed to fully awaken from anaesthesia for a smooth emergence unless intervention requires a deep extubation
- The incidence of laryngospasm is very high in this age group when awakening in a partially anaesthetized state. Suxamethonium 1–2mg/kg IV or 2–4mg/kg im, should be administered immediately and airway support given throughout
- The trachea should be extubated after the neonate is awake and meeting extubation criteria

Hyperactive airways/laryngospasm is commonly encountered in premature, ex-premature and term infants when their airways are manipulated.

Cases in which airway obstruction due to laryngospasm or bronchoconstriction ensues after induction are treated immediately with:

- 100% oxygen on positive pressure ventilation (PPV), if it does not resolve consider IV/IM suxamethonium
- Intubation with suxamethonium and support the cardiorespiratory system
- Beta 2 agonist puffs directly through the endotracheal tube if wheezing and bronchospasm ensues together with adding a volatile anaesthetic as a bronchodilator
- Orogastric suctioning to relieve intragastric pressure and ensure better ventilation
- Consider continued PPV with effective chest expansion avoiding volutrauma/barotrauma during the case and plan for transfer to a neonatal ICU postoperatively

Neonatal pain

In many instances we rely on behavioural changes and reactions of cry and facial activity to discriminate between non-invasive sensory events and pain provoked by an invasive procedure. Vital signs have been noted to change during manipulation of the eyes by ophthalmologists, especially during placement of eyelid speculums and the surgical procedure itself. We recommend:

- Tylenol rectal suppository 30–40mg/kg PR prior to surgical incision
- Applying anaesthetic eye drops immediately before speculum placement. Proparacaine hydrochlride 0.5% lasts 15min, tetracaine 0.5% can last up to 2h.
- Placing a peribulbar block at the end of the case (bupivacaine 0.25% at 50%volume with lidocaine 2% at 50% volume and total injectate volume per surgeon's discretion)

Once a neonate receives general anaesthesia, transportation to the NICU for further observation is the standard of care for infants with risks of apnoea of prematurity and or any other derangements that may warrant close observation of the patient in a monitored setting.

- Minimal traces of volatile anaesthetics can depress the hypoxic ventilatory response
- Hypoxia in itself will not stimulate but depress the respiratory drive
- All anaesthetics will reduce the functional residual capacity, which in turn is reflected as faster desaturations
- Infants are prone to airway obstruction and hyperactive airways; they have increased incidences of laryngospasm and bronchospasm

Avoiding delayed emergence and apnoea

- Refrain from the use of narcotics (unless warranted)
- Minimize muscle relaxation for intubation only
- Avoid conditions that would compromise a normal homeostatic environment for the infant

Electroretinography and multifocal electroretinography

Electroretinography and multifocal electroretinography

These examinations are widely used to test for retinal function, as a whole. The clinical preparation of the paediatric patient consists of:

- Maximum pupillary dilatation
- Pre-adaptation to darkness (20–30min)
- An area may be assigned to this adaptation or specially made black blinders are placed on the patient's eyes and the patient allowed to be held by the parent in the holding area
- Sedation/MAC vs. general anaesthesia
- Pre-exam sedation: this state of depressed consciousness is defined for three levels; minimal, moderate, and deep sedation. As the depth of sedation increases, protective airway reflexes may be compromised and ventilatory efforts decrease. Certain institutions are set up for electroretinography (ERG) to be performed outside the operating room in special dark rooms. After receiving a, the patient is appropriately monitored and allowed to reach a safe target sedative state and is placed supine for the ERG exam
- Facilities for assisting ventilation and administering oxygen are necessary adjuncts for all routes of administration of anaesthesia and sedation. Since cardiorespiratory arrest may occur, infants and children should be observed carefully during and after use of any sedative/ hypnotic and or opioid. Age- and size-appropriate resuscitative equipment (i.e., intubation and cardioversion equipment, oxygen, suction, and a secure intravenous line) and personnel qualified in its use must be immediately available
- An infant or child scheduled for GA for this exam may receive a preoperative sedative and without removing the blinders, undergo inhalation induction; an intravenous line is inserted and the patient is allowed to breathe spontaneously through an LMA or ETT. The operating room is darkened for the exam; the anaesthetist is permitted a red side light at his/her station. Infants and children undergoing ERG testing with general anaesthesia may have a more complete and comprehensive evaluation
- Sedatives are also used for ERG sedation
- Midazolam—oral 0.5–0.75mg/kg (up to 20mg):
  - Time of onset is 30–40min
  - Duration of effect is 60–90min
  - IV dose 0.05–0.2mg/kg
  - Rapid onset of action
  - Duration of effect is 45–60min
  - Reduce the doses by half if given with opioids
  - Simultaneous administration with opioids will give a synergistic effect and apnoea or prolonged sedation may occur
- Diazepam—IV 0.05–0.1mg/kg:
  - Onset of action is 5min
  - Duration of effect may be 60–120mins
- Temazepam—0.5–1mg/kg:
  - Oral solution comes in 10mg/5mls

Opioids
- Morphine oral solution 200–300mcg/kg:
  - Onset of action is 15–30 min
  - Duration of effect up to 2h
- Morphine IV dose 100–200 mcg/kg:
  - Onset of action is 10–15min
  - Reduce the dose if given with a benzodiazepine

Anaesthetic agents for sedation are used only by staff with training and experience in paediatric airway management, paediatric advanced life support (PALS) certified and all other contingencies that fall under the current policies for paediatric deep sedation at the institution responsible. Selection of appropriate drug and the correct dose is of paramount importance.

Cataract surgery

Glaucoma

Infantile glaucoma

Aberrant development of the trabecular mesh network with obstruction of flow of the aqueous humour causes infantile glaucoma. The classic triad of symptoms for congenital glaucoma includes tearing, photophobia, and blepharospasm. Infantile glaucoma develops within the first three years of life and is associated with:

- High intra-ocular pressure
- Enlargement of the eyes 'buphthalmic or ox-like' eyes
- Cloudy corneas
- Assessment of IOP is crucial to both diagnosis and determination of response to treatment
- Anaesthetic intervention introduces variables that may taint the accuracy of IOP measurements
- Normal range for IOP is 10–20mmHg
- All medications lower IOP in two main ways: decreasing the production of aqueous humour or by increasing its outflow from the eye

Children on medications

- Children may receive following medications:
  - Parasympathomimetics (e.g., pilocarpine):
    — Raises the aqueous humour outflow throughout the conventional route
    — Produces miosis and fall in IOP
    — Should be discontinued evening before surgery
    — Side effects rarely seen in children include diaphoresis, GI disturbances, hypotension and bradycardia
  - Miotics and sympathomimetics—epinephrine 0.5%, 1%, 2% (Epifrin® Allergan, Glaucon® Alcon), dipivefrin 0.1% (Propine® Allergan)
    — Decreases aqueous production by vasoconstriction within the ciliary body and in time desensitizes beta adrenergic response
    — Dipivefrin is an epinephrine prodrug with fewer side effects
    — Miotics do very little for infants because the muscle-tendon attachments that constrict the pupil and pull the iris are not well-developed
  - β-antagonists—timolol 0.25%–0.5% (Timoptic®Merck)
    — Suppresses aqueous humour formation
    — Least expensive
    — Common side effects seen: bradycardia, vertigo, bronchospasm and apnoea (Cheyne–Stokes breathing reported in neonates)
  - Betaxalol 0.5% (Betoptic® Alcon)
    — Cardioselective with less bronchial side effects
  - Timoptic XE® 0.25%–0.5% Merck
    — A gel solution with low concentrations
    — Preferred agent for paediatric glaucoma
    — Low systemic absorption

- Selective α2 agonists—brimonidine 0.15% and 2% (Alphagan P®
  Allergan)
  — Suppresses aqueous humour formation
  — Increases uveoscleral flow
  — Crosses the blood–brain barrier (BBB)
  — Relatively contraindicated in children
  — Side effects: somnolence, lethargy, CNS depression, apnoea
- Apradonidine 0.5%–1% (Lopidine® Alcon)
  — Less selective for the alpha receptors
  — Tachyphylaxis seen within 3 months
  — Useful for short-term treatment
- Carbonic anhidrase inhibitors—dorzolamide 2% (Trusopt® Merck)
  and Acetazolamide 1% (Azopt® Alcon)
  — Suppresses aqueous humour formation
  — Liquid suspension for paediatric use 8–30mg/kg/day
  — Side effects include anorexia, hyperpnoea, and urinary fre-
    quency
- Prostaglandin analogs—latanoprost 0.005% (Xalatan® Pfizer)
  Bimatoprost 0.03% (Lumigan® Allergan) Travaprost 0.004%
  (Travatan® Alcon) Unoprostone 0.155 (Rescula® Novartis)
  — Facilitates flow of aqueous humour via remodelling of the
    extracellular matrix of the uveoscleral path
  — Relaxes the ciliary muscle tone
  — Latanoprost has been used to treat older children
  — Juvenile-onset open-angle glaucoma and aphakic glaucoma in
    children have responded to treatment with latanoprost

Surgical treatment

Evaluation under anaesthesia

Measurements of the IOP are undertaken with a with a portable appla-
nation tonometer while the infant or child is breathing spontaneously in
stage III of a volatile anaesthetic with mixed O_2 and air or N_2O, commonly
used for induction in children. If surgery is decided, then insert an IV line
and the airway are secured with an LMA or ETT. Maintenance of anaesthesia is achieved with a balanced anaesthetic of a volatile agent mixed
with air and O_2, and low dose narcotics. Pre-emptive analgesia is achieved
with acetaminophen suppositories (30mg/kg) placed at the beginning of
the case. A peribulbar or sub-Tenon's block is performed by the surgeon
for postoperative pain coverage or anaesthetic eye drops placed.

Surgery

- Laser treatments: laser is directed towards the ciliary body to decrease
  its production of aqueous humour
- Goniotomy: an incision is made within the trabecular meshwork to
  allow for flow of the aqueous humour. To access this area and angle,
  the surgeon often needs to thin out the cornea for better view
- Trabeculotomy: this is the formation of a new drainage canal for the
  outflow of aqueous by placing a fine probe through Schlemm's canal
- Trabeculectomy: a new channel is formed for the outflow of aqueous
  humour from the anterior chamber to go into the sub-Tenon's space.
  The fluid is absorbed passively below the conjunctiva

Perioperative factors that affect IOP (see 📖 Intra-ocular pressure, pp. 40–43)

- Cerebral blood flow
- Venous pressure will usually equal IOP
- Increases in venous pressure increases IOP
- Coughing, straining, vomiting or valsalva decreases episcleral venous drainage
- Vasodilatation (hypercapnoea or use of carbonic anhydrase inhibitors) increases IOP due to less responsiveness or autoregulation distal to the central retinal artery
- Body/head position—on average there is a small change in pressure upon lying down, 0–2mmHg
- Anaesthetic drugs
- Narcotics, hypnotics, tranquillizers, volatile anaesthetics are associated with a decrease in IOP
- Ketamine does not decrease IOP
- Suxamethonium achieves a small, transient yet consistent rise in IOP of up to 7mmHg; induction agents may temper this
- General anaesthesia
- Airway management will increase IOP
- Intubation increases IOP as much as 30mmHg
- LMA can increase IOP by 2–3mmHg after uneventful placement
- The facemask may create apposition of trabecular meshwork to Schlemm's canal and elevate IOP
- Work of breathing under general anaesthesia is greater with a facemask and least with a tracheal tube
- Biometric measurement consideration with facemask vs. LMA vs. endotracheal tube
- Increased inspiratory pressures decrease IOP
- Insertion of an oral airway reduces inspiratory work of breathing
- Low pressure CPAP (5–6cm H_2O) with the LMA reduces inspiratory work of breathing
- Work of breathing with ETT is lower than facemask and LMA
- With respiratory fluctuations during quiet breathing there are 3mmHg of IOP fluctuation
- Measurement of IOP in children under general anaesthesia should be done prior to airway manipulation
- Preoperative dehydration decreases IOP
- Bell's phenomenon denotes light anaesthesia and may increase IOP or give false positives during tonometry

Effects of intraoperative regional anaesthesia

- The volume of LA used for retrobulbar and peribulbar injections may affect IOP. A peribulbar block provides adequate perioperative analgesia in all children. A regional anaesthetic allows reduction of anaesthetic requirements.

Postoperative pain

- Impact of pain on glaucoma eye surgery is mild. It can cause an increase in IOP postoperatively. An analgesic given during the surgery or in recovery should suffice

Strabismus surgery

Strabismus is a misalignment disorder of extra-ocular muscles characterized by amblyopia with or without anisometropia. The surgeon can distinguish between a paretic muscle and one that is restricted of movement by performing a forced duction test. This test is done under anaesthesia and the use a non-depolarizing muscle relaxant may be required in complex cases.

Strabismus may be inherited, developmental or acquired with or without associated comorbidities; particularly other neuromuscular disorders. It may not be uncommon for these children to have a hidden myopathy that will necessitate further investigation and prompt for perioperative precautions for a hypermetabolic reaction, malignant hyperpyrexia (MH) or masseter muscle spasm.

Anaesthetic technique

- Induction of general anaesthesia with inhalational or intravenous technique may follow with an LMA or a ETT. The patient is left on spontaneous ventilation with pressure support or intermittent positive pressure ventilation (IPPV)
- GA is maintained with a volatile anaesthetic mixed with air and O_2
- A TIVA may also reduce PONV in older children; it is not uncommon to administer an antiemetic as adjunctive therapy
- Antiemetics and analgesics are of value
- Muscle relaxation is not routinely indicated for non-complicated strabismus but in highly specialized practices, it may be required
- On-the-table traction test—a complex mutiplanar restrictive strabismus requires muscle relaxants to evaluate mechanical resistance of extra-ocular muscles (EOM) in absence of any EOM contraction.
  A slow tonic movement of both eyes may be seen after the conjunctiva is manipulated. This may interfere with the traction test and creates 'pseudo-restriction'. Deep anaesthesia or muscle relaxation may be required
- 'The fornix approach' to EOM surgery may require phenylephrine drops. Its absorption may be reduced by applying pressure against the tear ducts. It provides vasoconstriction and helps the surgeon identify anterior ciliary vessels. Dilation of the pupil helps in retinal visualization. Systemic effects of phenylephrine will produce a rise in blood pressure.

Oculo-cardiac reflex (see 📖 Oculo-cardiac reflex, pp. 44–45)

The ocular-cardiac reflex (OCR) is frequently encountered in children undergoing strabismus surgery.

- Attenuation of the OCR includes:
  - Pre-stimulus IV anticholinergics
  - Use of sevoflurane instead of halothane
  - Use of neuromuscular blocking drugs
  - Gentle surgical handling of the extra-ocular muscles
  - The OCR displays tachyphylaxis; repeated stimuli are often accompanied by attenuated responses

- First response to an OCR should be the cessation of surgical stimuli and simultaneous review of the patient's oxygenation, ventilation, and the depth of anaesthesia
- Compromising bradycardia with unstable haemodynamic requires the use of atropine

Hypermetabolic syndromes and EOM surgery

Strabismus may accompany a hidden myopathy and neuromuscular disorders that should alert clinicians to the incidence of masseter muscle rigidity (MMR), hypermetabolic disorders, and or MH when these children are exposed to triggering agents.

- This may range from 1 in 12000 for MMR to 1 in 100,000 for MH
- Clinical presentation of a hypermetabolic event under anaesthesia, the following signs are noted:
  - Elevation of CO_2 is the earliest and most sensitive sign specific to a hypermetabolic reaction
  - Tachycardia and tachypnoea: unfortunately infants normally present with increased sinus heart rates and the neuromuscular blocking (NMB) agents together with controlled ventilation offsets tachypnoea. Vigorous mask/bag ventilation may mask the rise of CO_2.
  - Blood pressure rises and presence of ventricular dysrrhythmias appear
  - Muscle tone increases
  - Body temperature increases 1–2° per every 5min or less.
  - The CO_2 absorbent becomes very warm
  - Peripheral mottling, sweating is noted without a marked decrease in oxygen saturation

A sample of mixed venous blood usually demonstrates ↑pCo_2, ↑K, ↑$Ca2^+$ and ↑lactic acid. CK levels usually surpass 20,000 units in 24 hours.

Masseter muscle spasm can be seen infrequently after the administration of suxamethonium, commonly in children and teenagers. It has also been seen to occur after the induction of anaesthesia with any volatile or IV anaesthetic.

Differential diagnosis include:

- Myotonic syndromes
- TMJ dysfunction
- Under dosing of suxamethonium and failing to allow an adequate circulation time for a dose of suxamethonium to reach effector sites
- Giving suxamethonium in the presence of increased resting tension of the skeletal muscle due to fever

Immediate management should consist of:

- Turning off the vaporizers
- Replacement of the anaesthesia circuit and machine and delivering 100% oxygen
- A call for the MH trolley or cart and alerting the team to begin cooling the patient
- Turn off all warming devices
- Force cooling of the patient with cold irrigates and ice packs
- Increase intravenous fluid administration and attain another peripheral IV site or central venous site

- Dantrolene mixed and given as per protocol
- An arterial or mixed venous gas sent out for gas analysis
- Cardiorespiratory support until the patient can be transferred to a PICU for further care and monitoring

Intraoperative hypermetabolic syndromes have deceased with:
- Improved identification of highly susceptible patients
- Avoidance of suxamethonium and other triggering agents
- Adhering to the department's policy for patients highly suspected of presenting a hypermetabolic event
- Use of total intravenous anaesthetics where warranted

Postoperative nausea and vomiting (PONV)

- There is an increased probability that the ocular-gastric reflex, mediated by the vagus nerve, be a response to surgical manipulation of the eye
- Diplopia may induce motion sickness and produce nausea and emesis
- Dehydration before surgery, electrolyte imbalances and prolonged stays in the recovery room are known to induce PONV in children after strabismus/ocular surgeries
- Strategies to minimize PONV:
  • Decreasing preoperative anxiety with benzodiazepines or clonidine
  • Propofol infusion-nitrous oxide technique (TIVA) reduces incidence and frequency of PONV
  • Avoid use of long-acting intraoperative narcotics (meperidine or morphine)
  • Tylenol 30–40mg/kg suppository or ketorolac 1mg/kg may be used as adjunct treatment

Peribulbar block or sub-Tenon's blocks with TIVA reduces incidence of PONV and consumption of analgesics. Postoperative analgesia and akinesia allows the surgical eye to adjust to visual axes alignment changes with a reduced incidence of vomiting.

Prophylaxis for PONV

The following drugs are known to reduce PONV:
- Avoid opioid analgesics
- Avoid nitrous oxide (controversial)
- IV dexamethasone 0.15–1mg/kg
- IV ondansetron 50–200mcg/kg
- IV metoclopramide 100–250mcg/kg

Emergency surgery and ophthalmic anaesthesia in the paediatric patient

The classification system for ocular trauma is very complex and readers are advised to read a specialist book on trauma.

Clinical assessment for the visual acuity in children presenting with trauma to the eye is attempted and documented if a child can communicate. A shield should be placed over the affected eye, especially if a laceration of the globe is suspected.

Open globe injuries in the pediatric population

Anterior segment globe injury—these lesions may be penetrating, with single full thickness lesions or perforating lesions with an entrance and exit wound.

Presence of an intra-ocular foreign object is not uncommon.

Lesions include:

- Superficial and conjunctival abrasions and lacerations
- Traumatic cataract
- Traumatic hyphaema
- Penetrating eye injuries

Anaesthetic technique

In a fasted child with no IV in place:

- A preoperative sedative may be administered via oral route. Attempts to place an IV preoperatively may precipitate crying and squeezing of the eyelids that may increase IOP up to 70mmHg
- A gentle inhalation based induction is performed and IV placed. Skilled personnel should attempt IV access prior to intubation
- Airway is secured appropriately considering unpredicted duration of surgery

Child with suspected full stomach:

- Preparation for a rapid sequence induction (RSI) is undertaken when a delay in surgery carries an increased risk to the patient's visual outcome
- EUA with general anaesthesia for primary surgical intention: the goal is to secure an airway with minimal risks of aspiration
- During the RSI, all anaesthesia personnel must be ready to bag/mask ventilate the infant or child and perform immediate intubation
- Suxamethonium is avoided when extrusion of intra-ocular contents is imminent with minor changes of IOP
- Measures to prevent secondary haemorrhage and/or corneal blood staining
- Contraindications to RSI include infants and children with known airway anomalies or facial anomalies in which placement of an endotracheal tube may be difficult or impossible and in which succession of spontaneous respirations may be potentially lethal
- Consider analgesic coverage for deep extubation and a smooth emergence after the patient meets all extubation criteria

Emergence delirium in children

Emergence from general anaesthesia is defined as a smooth transition through the four stages of anaesthesia to a fully awake state. In less than 10% of surgical cases, delirium on emergence may ensue and compromise the surgical site and extend post-anaesthesia recovery time. This is described as a period of restlessness, agitation, and disorientation. Screaming, kicking, and yelling may occur.

Physiologic causes

- Hypoxaemia
- Hypercapnoea
- Respiratory depression
- Pain
- Hypothermia
- Electrolyte imbalance
- Sensory deprivation
- Sensory overload

Pharmacologic causes

- Central anticholinergic syndrome (atropine and scopolamine)
- Residual effects of anaesthetics
- Droperidol
- Metroclopramide
- Benzodiazepines
- Narcotics
- Ketamine
- Atropine

Treatment

- Rule out physiologic and pharmacologic reasons
- Supplemental oxygen
- Electrolyte replacement
- Analgesics
- Physostigmine 0.02mg/kg IM or IV slowly, will reverse delirium caused by anticholinergics
- Naloxone (®Narcan) 0.01mg/kg IV, IM or subcutaneously (SC) may be given for opioid induced respiratory depression
- Flumazenil (®Romazicon) 0.01mg/kg IV may be given over 15min to reverse sedation due to benzodiazepines

Conclusion

There are a plethora of anaesthesia considerations for the neonate, infant, or child undergoing ophthalmologic surgery. The anaesthetist must be knowledgeable about apnoea, the particular ramifications of the oculocardiac reflex in this population, postoperative nausea and vomiting and more, in addition to the standard issues for adults having eye surgery.

Key reading

Pun MS, Thakur J, Gurung R. Ketamine anesthesia for pediatric ophthalmology surgery. *Br. J. Ophthalmology*. 2003; 87: 535–77.

Sihota R, Tuli D, Dada T. Distribution and determinants of IOP in normal pediatric distribution. *Journal Pediatric Ophthalmology Strabismus*. 2006; 43: 14–18.

Chapter 14

Anaesthesia for glaucoma surgery

Mr Tom Eke

Introduction

'Glaucoma' is a term used to describe a group of sight-threatening eye conditions, which may need surgery to reduce the intra-ocular pressure (IOP). High IOP is caused by impaired circulation of aqueous humour in the anterior segment of the eyeball (see 📖 Intra-ocular pressure, p. 40). High IOP (or poor blood supply) can damage the axons of the optic nerve and cause gradual visual loss, usually over the course of many months or years. Axonal damage occurs at the optic nerve head, where the nerve exits the globe. Peripheral vision is affected first, so glaucoma may not be noticed until vision loss is advanced. Lost vision cannot be restored, but lowering the IOP reduces the risk of further sight loss. Extremely high IOP can cause sudden visual loss, often by occlusion of the central retinal artery.

Classification of glaucoma

Acute versus chronic glaucoma

There are several ways of categorizing the glaucomas:
- An acute rise in IOP usually presents as a painful (aching) red eye with reduced vision. The cornea may be hazy and the eyeball feels hard
- Chronic glaucoma is more common. It is usually diagnosed when asymptomatic, during a spectacles check. Advanced cases may present with painless worsening of peripheral vision, over many months

Open-angle vs. narrow/closed-angle glaucoma

- Open angle means that the anterior chamber drainage angle (between iris and cornea) is open. In the commonest type of open-angle glaucoma, aqueous humour can reach the angle, but drainage is impaired at the level of the trabecular meshwork, within the angle itself
- Narrow angle occurs in smaller eyes, as the lens continues to grow with normal ageing. If the lens grows too large for the eye, the angle may close completely. This may cause acute or chronic glaucoma
- In predisposed eyes, anti-muscarinic agents (e.g. atropine, scopolamine) can induce acute angle closure glaucoma

High IOP vs. 'low tension' or 'normal pressure' glaucoma

- Classically, glaucoma was considered to be simply due to high IOP causing damage to the optic nerve. High IOP is due to impaired drainage of aqueous humour (hypersecretion is exceedingly rare)
- Glaucoma may also occur despite normal measured IOP, because of:
  - Thin cornea causing underestimation of true IOP
  - Variable IOP (e.g. high IOP in mornings, but measured in afternoon)
  - Large diurnal swings in IOP (diagnose with a day of hourly IOPs)
  - Poor blood supply to optic nerve head: low BP or nocturnal dips in BP, vasospasm, Raynaud's, migraine, etc.
  - Masquerade syndrome (e.g. optic nerve infarct, pituitary tumour)
- Additional treatments for 'true low-tension glaucoma' may include:
  - Calcium antagonists (e.g. nifidipine)
  - Herbal extracts (e.g. ginkgo biloba, which affects bleeding times)

Surgical procedures in glaucoma

Surgical procedures in glaucoma

Trabeculectomy

The 'standard' glaucoma surgical procedure is known as trabeculectomy (see Figure 14.1). A small hole is made in the sclera, to allow the aqueous humour to drain more freely to the conjunctival veins (trabeculectomy). Typical surgery time is 20–60min. Common standard steps are:

- Stay suture to pull eye downward (risks of oculo-cardiac reflex)
- Superior conjunctiva and Tenon's capsule reflected
- Diathermy to sclera, to minimize bleeding
- Scleral flap, making a 'trapdoor' above the limbus
- Entry into anterior chamber, peripheral iridectomy
- Suturing of scleral flap, conjunctiva
- Topical antimetabolite (e.g. mitomicin, 5-fluorouracil) reduces scarring

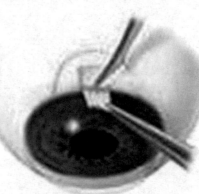

Fig. 14.1 Penetrating trabeculectomy.

The main reason for failure is over-healing of Tenon's layer.

Anticoagulants/antiplatelets are usually stopped for 1–3 weeks (risk of sight-threatening choroidal haemorrhage if initial low IOP).

Non-penetrating trabeculectomy (viscocanalostomy, deep sclerectomy)

Steps are similar to trabeculectomy, but no hole is made into the anterior chamber. There is less risk of hypotony but long-term IOP control less good.

Glaucoma drainage device (tubes and shunts)

Surgical steps are similar to trabeculectomy, but a tube or shunt is inserted into the anterior chamber, under the scleral flap (see Figures 14.2 to 14.6). The tube is attached to a plate, which is sutured to the sclera, and covered with Tenon's and conjunctiva.

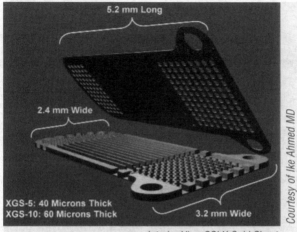

Fig. 14.2 Gold shunt.

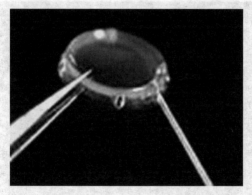

Fig. 14.3 Moltano tube.

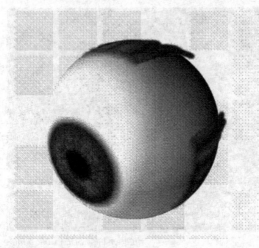

Fig. 14.4 Ahmed tube.

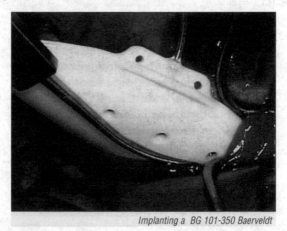

Implanting a BG 101-350 Baerveldt

Fig. 14.5 Baerveldt device.

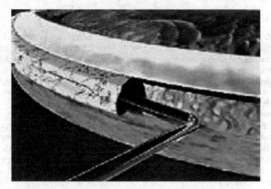

Fig. 14.6 Viscacalastomy procedure.

Cataract surgery and glaucoma

Cataract is common in glaucoma patients, partly due to eye drops and surgery. Cataract surgery may 'cure' a narrow drainage angle. Postoperative inflammation may cause a previous glaucoma operation to fail. Increasingly combined glaucoma and cataract surgery are performed.

Cycloablation (cyclo-diode laser, cyclo-cryotherapy)

Ablation of the ciliary body makes the eye produce less aqueous humour, thus reducing IOP. The procedure is quick and easy for the patient, but there is a higher risk of hypotony and retinal oedema. Good analgesia is needed. There is no need to stop anticoagulant/antiplatelet agents.

Anaesthesia for glaucoma surgery

Trabeculectomy surgery is performed both under general or any of the local regional anaesthesia techniques (📖 see Chapters 6, 7, & 8). Local anaesthesia (LA) can be either placed behind the globe (intraconal/retrobulbar, extraconal/peribulbar or posterior sub-Tenon's blocks) or at front of globe (subconjunctival, anterior sub-Tenon's, topical or intracameral).

Risk of visual loss from anaesthesia

Sight-threatening and life-threatening complications of GA and LA are discussed elsewhere (📖 see Chapters 11, 12, & 21). Many sight-threatening complications occur at the level of the optic nerve or optic nerve head. In glaucoma, the optic nerve is already damaged and may be more vulnerable to pressure or ischaemic insult. This means that glaucomatous eyes may be at higher risk of visual loss if a sight-threatening complication does occur.

Specific concerns in glaucoma patients are:
- Higher risk of visual loss, if a 'sight-threatening' complication occurs
- 'Wipe-out' of vision
- Failure of trabeculectomy (return to high IOP)

Wipe-out of vision in glaucoma patients

Wipe-out of visual field means total loss of vision in the eye after surgery, with no obvious cause. Some studies give an incidence as high as 1–2%. Eyes with pre-existing glaucomatous field defects appear to be at higher risk. Total loss is called 'wipe-out' or 'snuff syndrome', but less severe cases may present as unexplained worsening of visual field. Often, with time, vision returns.

If there is no obvious cause, probable aetiologies relate to intrinsic optic nerve status, surgical factors, and/or postoperative alterations in IOP. Anaesthesia-related mechanisms have not been proven. Postulated theoretical anaesthesia factors include:
- LA puts pressure on an already compromised/vulnerable optic nerve:
  - Mass effect or compartment syndrome (LA trapped in fascial compartment behind globe)
  - Pressure device used after LA
  - Retrobulbar haemorrhage
  - Hyaluronidase orbitopathy
- Direct trauma to optic nerve:
  - Needle damage to optic nerve
  - Haematoma of optic nerve
- Hypoperfusion of optic nerve head:
  - Pressure/trauma, as above
  - Vasoconstrictor mixed with LA mix (e.g. epinephrine)
  - Low blood pressure (with GA)
  - Trauma to posterior ciliary vessels (posterior sub-Tenon's block)

Failure of trabeculectomy

The commonest cause of trabeculectomy failure is scarring of Tenon's layer and conjunctiva. This may occur at any time following surgery. Risk factors include prior trauma (including surgery), which primes the conjunctival fibroblasts to induce scar tissue. It would be logical to infer that chemosis or subconjunctival haemorrhage, caused by LA, might therefore increase the risk of trabeculectomy failure. This could apply to a past, present, or future trabeculectomy. There is some evidence that lidocaine may have a direct inhibitory effect on conjunctival fibroblasts, analogous to the antimetabolites, which might reduce the risk of failure.

At present the literature is insufficient to support the above assertions. A few (small) prospective randomized trials have compared different LA techniques for trabeculectomy, with no significant effect on IOP control. Thus, it appears that anaesthesia technique does not have a major influence on the outcome of trabeculectomy. No studies have looked at whether anaesthesia technique for cataract surgery might affect the outcome of a future trabeculectomy, or an existing trabeculectomy.

Suggested anaesthesia techniques for specific procedures

Trabeculectomy, non-penetrating surgery and tube implants

- Any GA or LA technique can be used
- Avoid LA mass effect behind eye (risk of wipe-out, 📖 see Wipe-out of vision in glaucoma patients, p. 230)
- Avoid use of decompression devices
- Best to discuss with surgeon first!
- This author prefers subconjunctival or intracameral LA (no risk of wipe-out, quick and easy, possible improved IOP control)

Cyclo-ablation (cyclo-diode and cyclo-cryotherapy)

- GA or LA placed behind globe gives best analgesia
- Subconjunctival LA can be used, but LA must be given time to work
- Topical LA insufficient
- This author prefers small-volume posterior sub-Tenon's LA as it is quick, provides excellent analgesia with little chemosis. The retained eye movements make procedure simple

Cataract surgery in glaucoma patients

- Any GA or LA technique can be used
- Avoid LA mass effect behind eye (risk of wipe-out, 📖 see Wipe-out of vision in glaucoma patients, p. 230)
- This author prefers topical and/or intracameral LA (no risk of haemorrhage/chemosis which might affect past/future trabeculectomy function)

Special anaesthesia techniques

Most glaucoma surgery can be done using the standard GA or LA techniques. Many glaucoma surgeons have a preferred technique, so surgeon and anaesthesiologist should discuss this. General and various regional anaesthesia techniques are discussed elsewhere (see Chapters 11 & 12). In this section, the author's preferred techniques other than regional techniques are described in detail.

Subconjunctival and intracameral LA

This is a quick efficient technique, with good patient satisfaction. The LA can be given when the patient arrives in the operating room, and there is no delay in waiting for the LA to take effect. The author uses non-preserved lidocaine 0.5% for both subconjunctival and intracameral LA. Others may use different strengths (e.g. 2% lidocaine with epinephrine subconjunctival, 1% lidocaine intracameral).

- Topical anaesthesia and povidone iodine drops before LA is given
- Subconjunctival LA under operating microscope
  - Less risk of haemorrhage as larger vessels can be avoided
  - Ask patient to look downward, warn that LA may sting a little
- Sub-conjunctival injection of about 0.5ml lidocaine, using fine needle
  - Injection to cover area of proposed bleb
  - If LA does not spread properly, can massage through the eyelid
- No stay suture is needed, as patient is asked to 'look down' for surgery
- Additional topical tetracaine 1% to bare sclera, prior to diathermy
- Intracameral LA before peripheral iridectomy
- No stay suture makes scleral/conjunctival suturing easier

Topical and intracameral LA

Clear-corneal approach to phacoemulsification is particularly suited to glaucoma patients, as it avoids the conjunctiva and Tenon's layer (thus maintaining trabeculectomy function).

- Patient is counselled before surgery
  - Expect some awareness of surgery
  - They may see shadows, swirling lights, or may lose light perception
- Proxymetacaine, povidone-iodine drops to start
- Additional LA drops (e.g tetracaine) optional
- Clear-corneal incision
- Non-preserved lidocaine 0.5% or 1% to anterior chamber
- Patient is reminded to look towards the light of operating microscope:
  - This keeps the eye 'on axis' for easier surgery
  - If patient finds light too bright, turn it down then gradually brighten

Examination under general anaesthesia for glaucoma

Examination under anaesthesia (EUA) is occasionally needed for glaucoma patients (see Ophthalmic evaluations under anaesthesia in premature children, p.206–207). The most common scenario is congenital glaucoma, requiring multiple EUA's over many years for the purposes of diagnosis and IOP monitoring. The main concern is to avoid doing anything that might significantly alter the intra-ocular pressure (IOP) during GA (see Chapter 3, pp. 42–43).

- Ketamine has minimal effect on IOP
- LMA has minimal effect on IOP
- Depolarizing neuromuscular blocking agent will cause transient IOP rise
- Pressure from facemask may raise IOP
- Many agents and manoeuvres have an effect on IOP

For children who will require multiple EUA's for IOP monitoring purposes, it is usually best to use a consistent GA technique for each EUA that the patient undergoes. This should minimize the effect of minor variations in technique on the IOP and enables the paediatric glaucoma specialist to compare serial IOP measurements.

Systemic problems from glaucoma medications

Glaucoma patients are usually treated with topical medication (eye-drops) or oral medication to lower IOP. Eye drops will also enter the circulation: thus they may cause systemic side effects and drug interactions. Some of these can be life-threatening. Common and important associations are given here. For the full list, see datasheets for each medication.

Beta-adrenoceptor blockers (beta-blockers)

Eye drops: timolol, carteolol, betaxolol, levobunolol, etc. Very commonly used as eye-drops to treat chronic glaucoma. Many 'combination' glaucoma drops include timolol with another agent. Systemic absorption and systemic side effects are common. Oral beta-blockers do reduce IOP, but not used clinically for this.

- Contraindicated: asthma (exacerbation of bronchospasm):
  - The 'cardioselective' betaxolol may also exacerbate asthma
- Contraindicated: bradycardia, heart block, uncontrolled heart failure
- Numerous drug interactions, e.g. verapamil (hypotension, asystole)
- Systemic side effects common, including:
  - Bronchospasm, bradycardia, hypotension, peripheral vasoconstriction, fatigue, headache
- Caution in diabetes:
  - May interfere with metabolic/autonomic response to hypoglycemia

Prostaglandin analogues

Eye drops: latanoprost, bimatoprost, travoprost, tafluprost, etc. These are very commonly used as eye drops to treat chronic glaucoma.
- Systemic side effects are rare
- Very rarely, chest pain or exacerbation of angina

Carbonic anhydrase inhibitors

- Oral: acetazolamide tablets (usually short-term, for days or weeks)
- Eye drops: dorzolamide, brinzolamide
- Intravenous: acetazolamide (emergency IOP lowering)
- Commonly used as eye drops to treat chronic glaucoma
- Acetazolamide may be used to reduce IOP prior to surgery
- Frequent side effects with systemic administration
- Serious systemic effects rare with topical administration
- Acetazolamide has diuretic effect
- Electrolyte disturbance with prolonged systemic use
- Metabolic acidosis with systemic use
- Sulphonamide-related side effects and sensitivity
- Acetazolamide contraindicated if:
  - Hypokalemia, hyponatremia, hyperchloremic acidosis
  - Renal impairment, severe hepatic impairment
  - Sulphonamide hypersensitivity

Sympathomimetics, alpha-adrenergic agonists

Eye drops: brimonidine, apraclonidine, adrenaline, dipivefrine.
- Brimonidine commonly used as eye-drops to treat chronic glaucoma
- Apraclonidine commonly used as pre-treatment prior to surgery
- May cause hypertension, palpitations, syncope
- Interaction with monoamine oxidase inhibitor (MAOI) (hypertension risk)

Parasympathomimetics/muscarinic agonists

Eye drops: pilocarpine
- Uncommon in modern practice as treatment for chronic glaucoma
- Often used to treat acute angle closure
- May be used as pre-treatment before surgery (e.g trabeculectomy)
- Systemic side effects rare with eye drops
- Caution in cardiac disease, hypertension, asthma, peptic ulceration, urinary tract obstruction, Parkinson's
- May cause bronchospasm, bradycardia, diarrhoea, urinary retention

Osmotic diuretics

Oral: glycerol e.g. 1.5g/kg bodyweight orally, with fruit juice
- Intravenous: mannitol e.g. 20%, up to 500ml slow IV
- For emergency reduction of IOP: may be used just prior to surgery:
  - Diuresis causes full bladder, surgical patient may be uncomfortable
  - Contraindicated in severe cardiac failure, pulmonary oedema, dehydration, anuria
  - Caution with renal impairment, monitor fluid/electrolyte balance
- Side effects include hypotension, thrombophlebitis, fluid/electrolyte imbalance, arrhythmias, hypertension, pulmonary oedema, urinary retention, dehydration; rarely heart failure, renal failure etc.

Cholinesterase inhibitors

Eye drops: phospholine Iodide (echothiopate)
- Rarely/never used, but still available in some countries (not UK):
  - High-risk respiratory/cardiovascular collapse with GA
  - 'Suxamethonium apnoea'

Stopping antiplatelet and anticoagulant medication

Glaucoma surgery may cause a period of hypotony (low IOP), which puts the eye at risk of a sight-threatening haemorrhage from the choroid. To minimize likelihood, many surgeons will discontinue anticoagulant or antiplatelet medication for some days or weeks around the time of surgery.

Acute glaucoma occurring during anaesthesia in patients undergoing non-glaucoma procedures

Acute IOP rise can occasionally occur in patients who have surgery for unrelated glaucoma problems. It should not occur in patients who are known to have a glaucoma diagnosis, because their ophthalmologist will have done some prophylactic treatment (usually a laser iridotomy). If there is any suspicion of acute IOP rise, an ophthalmologist should be consulted urgently. Prompt diagnosis and treatment usually saves the sight.

Clinical features of acute glaucoma in suspected cases
- Painful (aching) eye
- Blurred vision (hazy, sometimes with rainbow haloes around lights)
- Red eye (redness mainly around the cornea)
- Globe feels hard to touch
- Cornea may appear hazy, pupil usually dilated
- Nausea, vomiting, abdominal pain:
  - Occasionally, this is the major feature and the patient may be mis-diagnosed to have an acute abdominal problem

Acute angle closure glaucoma (acute primary angle closure)
This is the commonest cause of acute glaucoma, including postoperative acute glaucoma. It occurs because of a combination of:
- Small globe (hypermetropic, or 'long-sighted' eye)
- Enlarging lens (due to ageing, pushes iris forward)
- Dilated pupil (e.g. caused by pain, dim light, medications):
  - E.g antimuscarinics: atropine, scopolamine, etc.

At risk patients
- Older age (60s and above)
- Hypermetropic:
  - Wears 'magnifying' spectacles which make the eyes look larger
  - Without spectacles/contact lenses, vision is blurred for near and far
- Not under the care of an ophthalmologist
- Prone positioning for surgery
- Anterior chamber of eye looks shallow, as big lens pushes iris forward:
  - Illuminate the eyeball using a pen-torch, with the torch held at the side, in the plane of the pupil
  - In a normal eye, all of the iris will be illuminated
  - If the anterior chamber is shallow, the nasal part of the iris will be in shadow. You will have to move the torch forward in order to illuminate the entire iris
  - If in doubt, ask an ophthalmologist

Acute glaucoma caused by GA after vitreoretinal surgery (expansion of intra-ocular gas bubble)

Some vitreoretinal operations involve putting a bubble of gas inside the eyeball, in order to hold the retina in place (see 📖 Physiologic principles, pharmacologic agents, and techniques of general anaesthesia, p. 176–177 and Vitrectomy, p. 244). Typical indications include macular hole surgery and some retinal detachment procedures. Gases are typically perfluoro-carbons such as sulfur hexafluoride (SF_6) or octafluoropropane (C_3F_8). Long-acting bubbles may stay in the eye for some weeks after surgery. These bubbles will expand to several times their original volume when exposed to nitrous oxide. Thus, if a patient has another GA in the weeks following this type of surgery, nitrous oxide will cause gas bubble to expand, causing high IOP and blindness due to retinal arterial occlusion. The patient may complain of a painful eye in the recovery area, but the vision may have already been lost.

Steps to avoid this problem
- Anaesthetists should be aware of this risk, and ask patients for details about recent surgery prior to giving GA
- If patient needs a further GA in the weeks following insertion of a gas bubble, nitrous oxide should not be given until it is certain that the bubble has completely resolved
- During vitreoretinal surgery under GA, the anaesthetist should turn off nitrous oxide, well before the gas-bubble is inserted
- Patients should be warned about this risk
- Patients given a wristband to wear, in case emergency surgery is needed. Gas manufacturers now provide these warning wristbands
- If acute glaucoma is suspected, the patient will need urgent assessment by an ophthalmologist. Untreated, acute glaucoma is likely to lead to permanent blindness. Prompt assessment and treatment will usually save the eyesight

Conclusion

A careful pre-assessment of patients undergoing glaucoma surgery is essential. An understanding of physiology of IOP, drugs affecting the IOP and how these changes can be minimized is of paramount importance. Anaesthesia technique varies from GA, regional ophthalmic anaesthesia and topical anaesthesia. The choice of anaesthesia depends on the complex medical condition of the patient, surgical procedure for glaucoma surgery and preference of the surgeon.

Key reading

Eke T. Anaesthesia for glaucoma surgery. *Current Anaesthesia & Critical Care.* 2010; 21(4): 168–73.

Khaw PT, Shah P, Elkington AR. Glaucoma 1: diagnosis. *Br. Med. J.* 2004; 328: 97–9.

Khaw PT, Shah P, Elkington AR. Glaucoma 2: treatment. *Br. Med. J.* 2004; 328: 156–8.

Anaesthesia for vitreoretinal surgery

Dr Joanna Budd

Dr K.-L. Kong

Introduction

Vitreoretinal (VR) surgery involves the management of vitreous and retinal diseases of the eye. Evolution of surgical techniques over the past 30 years has been significant, allowing many more procedures to be done as day cases under regional anaesthesia with monitored anaesthesia care. Conditions presenting for VR surgery are varied and are managed with essentially two types of operation: the vitrectomy, where the vitreous and retina are approached internally, and the scleral buckle procedure, which uses an external approach.

Conditions presenting for VR surgery

- Vitreous haemorrhage can lead to a profound reduction of vision. It often accompanies disorders of the retina and common causes include diabetic retinopathy and retinal vein occlusion. It can be successfully treated by vitrectomy
- Retinal detachment is where the retina detaches from the underlying retinal pigment epithelium
- Rhegmatogenous retinal detachment (detachment with holes) occurs due to a tear or hole in the retina that allows fluid from the vitreous cavity to pass into the subretinal space
- Other types of detachment include exudative, where fluid accumulates under the retina from inflammation, injury or a vascular abnormality without a hole or tear, and tractional, where fibrovascular tissue arising from trauma or neovascularization pulls the retina from the pigment epithelium. Retinal detachment is more common in severely myopic eyes and there is an increased risk of detachment after cataract surgery
- Urgent surgery is required in those patients in whom the macula is still attached at the time of presentation or where subretinal fluid is likely to extend rapidly
- Surgical treatment includes cryobuckle surgery and vitrectomy with the use of a gas bubble or silicone oil to tamponade the retina. Once the macula has detached visual outcomes do not change provided that the operation is performed within seven days post-detachment
- Retinal detachments that have been present for some time may be complicated by proliferative vitreoretinopathy. Surgical treatment for this may include retinopexy, a process of forming chorioretinal adhesions around the torn part of the retina
- Diabetic eye disease may result in vitreous haemorrhage or tractional retinal detachment
- Trauma to the eye can result in a number of conditions necessitating VR surgery. These include dislocation of the lens, retinal detachment, and vitreous haemorrhage as well as intra-ocular foreign bodies such as metal fragments. Urgency of surgery is dependent of the type of injury with penetrating injuries requiring more immediate repair
- Complications of cataract surgery may require VR surgery. The lens may dislocate into the vitreous during phacoemulsification ('dropped nucleus') which requires urgent vitrectomy. Postoperative endophthalmitis may be managed with vitreous biopsy and intra-vitreal injection of antibiotics. Globe perforation from sharp needles, rigid sub-Tenon's cannulae, or scissors used with regional anaesthetic techniques may cause choroidal or vitreous haemorrhage and tears in the retina can result in retinal detachment. Injection of local anaesthetic directly into the eye may lead to scleral rupture

VR surgical procedures

Vitrectomy

This is the most commonly performed VR operation involving an internal approach to the vitreous and retina, with removal of some or all of the vitreous. It is generally done under regional anaesthesia as there is no traction on the external ocular muscles and painful pulling does not occur. It involves the placement of three holes in the sclera for insertion of an infusion cannula, a light source and the surgical instrument (see Figure 15.1). The vitreous and retina are viewed through a dilated pupil using a wide angle indirect viewing system attached to the operating microscope. The surgeon is able to examine and treat the retina directly.

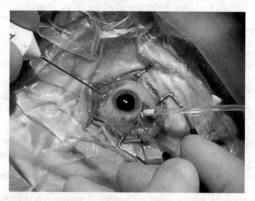

Fig. 15.1 Various ports during vitrectomy.

Vitrectomy is used in the treatment of many conditions such as retinal detachment, vitreous haemorrhage, diabetic retinopathy, macula pucker, and macula holes. It is also used in the management of ocular trauma and infection. Internal tamponade of the retina with gases or silicone oils is commonly used during this procedure. Tamponading prevents accumulation of fluid through a break in the retina and forces the retina outwards. Common gases used are sulfahexafluoride (SF_6) and perfluoropropane (C_3F_8) diluted with air in a non-expansile concentration. These are gradually reabsorbed, SF_6 within 10 days of surgery and C_3F_6 within six weeks. If used undiluted they expand to twice (SF_6) or four times (C_3F_8) their volume postoperatively. Patients with gas bubbles *in situ* should be warned about the risks of flying, where decreases in cabin pressure cause the bubble to expand, and general anaesthesia using nitrous oxide (see 📖 Physiologic principles, pharmacologicagents, and techniques of general anaesthesia pp. 176–177 and Acute glaucoma caused by GA after vitreoretinal surgery (expansion of intraocular gas bubble) p. 239). Originally, ophthalmic surgeons believed that patients needed to be in prone position during initial placement of the intra-ocular gas (see Fig. 15.2 and Fig. 15.3). The gas was instilled following surgery but prior to emergence from anaesthesia, thus requiring moving the anaesthetized patient from supine to prone position. Silicone oil is used when more permanent tamponade is required and needs to be removed at a later date.

Scleral buckle surgery

This is used for the treatment of retinal detachments and may be done under GA or RA. Traction on the globe during this procedure can stimulate the oculo-cardiac reflex and may be painful if there is inadequate anaesthesia. Slings are placed round the recti muscles to facilitate traction of the globe. The indirect ophthalmoscope is used to look for retinal breaks, which can then be treated by cryotherapy applied externally. A silicone sponge or solid explant is sutured to the sclera and subretinal fluid may be drained. The explant pushes the wall of the globe towards the retinal break allowing the retina to reattach. Intra-ocular pressure (IOP) may rise as the sutures around the explant are tightened. If the IOP rises above 70mmHg the central artery of the retina may be occluded.

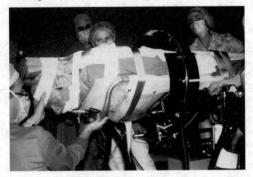

Fig. 15.2 Originally, ophthalmic surgeons believed that patients needed to be in prone position during initial placement of the intra-ocular gas. It was instilled following surgery but prior to emergence from anaesthesia, thus requiring moving the anaesthetized patient from supine to prone position (Courtesy Bascom Palmer Eye Institute Photographic Archives).

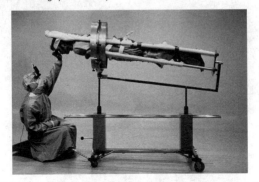

Fig. 15.3 Historical photo of patient in prone position, readied for injection of intra-vitreal agent. (Courtesy Bascom Palmer Eye Institute Photographic Archives).

Choice of anaesthetic technique

Traditionally, the chosen method of anaesthesia for VR surgery was general anaesthesia as the procedures were thought to be too long and potentially too uncomfortable for patients to be able to tolerate whilst awake. However, in the past 10 years there has been a growing trend for VR procedures to be done very successfully under RA with MAC. This trend has followed that which occurred with cataract surgery. Day-case VR operations have become feasible with improvements in surgical equipment and techniques given that safe and effective LA blocks are available. RA for VR surgery has some major advantages over GA.

These include:
• Faster recovery and the ability to perform VR procedures as day cases
• Minimal metabolic interference (e.g. diabetic patients and those on dialysis)
• Superior postoperative analgesia
• Partial or complete blockade of the oculo-cardiac reflex
• Reduced postoperative nausea and vomiting
• Immediate commencement of postoperative posturing where required

There may be some circumstances where RA is less ideal and GA is the preferred choice, particularly in younger patients and those undergoing more complex surgery. Some believe that general anaesthesia may also be preferable when the VR procedure is being done on the patient's only eye as local anaesthesia may render the eye sightless due to a temporary effect on the optic nerve, and an anaesthetized eye is more prone to injury. In some patients who have had scleral buckle surgery, spread of LA agents around the eye can be limited by scar tissue and it may not be possible to get good anaesthesia with LA alone.

In practice the choice of anaesthetic technique is largely governed by the general health of the patient and the preferences of both the patient and clinicians.

Preoperative assessment and preparation

Many patients undergoing VR surgery are older and have associated medical conditions such as diabetes, therefore careful preoperative assessment is necessary especially when considering GA (⬚ see Chapters 5 & 11). As well as a medical assessment, the preoperative preparation should include a full explanation of the procedure, discussion of the alternative anaesthesia modalities, explanation about the length of surgery and the implications this will have for the patient if the procedure is being done under RA.

Investigations

With regard to ophthalmic patients, no routine screening tests have been shown to be helpful or to improve outcome. The Joint Royal Colleges' Guidelines on local anaesthesia for intra-ocular surgery (2001) recommends that tests should only be considered when the patient history or findings on physical examination would have indicated the need for an investigation even if surgery had not been planned. The blood sugar in diabetic patients should be controlled and the international normalized ratio (INR) may be checked in those patients on warfarin.

When VR surgery under GA is considered, it is desirable for eye units to develop local protocols regarding preoperative investigations to ensure consistency and minimize any disruption to patient care. In the UK, most units have adopted recommendations published by NICE in 2003.

Patients on anticoagulants and antiplatelet medications

It is common to find that patients presenting for VR surgery are on aspirin, warfarin or clopidogrel. These are prescribed to reduce the incidence of thromboembolic events in patients with cardiovascular disease but they could potentially lead to orbital haemorrhage in patients undergoing eye surgery.

There have been no randomized controlled trials undertaken to address the risks and benefits of anticoagulants and antiplatelet drugs during ophthalmic surgery. However, observational studies have found that it was safe to continue with these agents during the perioperative period in patients having VR surgery without a higher incidence of potentially sight-threatening LA or operative haemorrhagic complications and suggest that no change in ongoing anticoagulants or antiplatelet drugs is necessary. For those on warfarin, the Joint Colleges' advice is that the INR should be checked and this should be within the recommended therapeutic ratio determined by the condition for which the patient is being anticoagulated. Others question the utility of obtaining an INR if the intention is to proceed with surgery regardless of the result. Where there are any specific concerns (e.g. complicated surgery or only eye surgery), there should be discussion between clinicians and patients regarding the risks and benefits of continuing anticoagulants and antiplatelet drugs to agree an acceptable approach.

Regional anaesthesia techniques

The ideal conditions provided by any RA technique for eye surgery are globe and conjunctival anaesthesia, globe and lid akinesia, and a soft eye with normal or reduced intra-ocular pressure. VR surgical procedures take longer and are potentially more stimulating than small-incision phacoemulsification for cataract surgery. This is particularly true of cryo-buckling procedures. In addition good akinesia is more important for certain VR procedures such as membrane peeling. The LA block therefore needs to be of sufficient depth and duration of action to allow for this.

Although topical anaesthesia has been used for shorter and less complicated VR operations with transconjunctival sutureless 23 or 25 gauge instruments, the eye remains fully mobile and anaesthesia may not be adequate enough to prevent pain on scleral puncture and patients may require additional sedation or analgesia. Retrobulbar techniques are now rarely used in the UK due to the recognized sight- and life-threatening complications. Peribulbar and sub-Tenon's techniques provide excellent operating conditions and are commonly employed.

Choice and dose of local anaesthetic agent

Lidocaine 2% has a rapid onset of action but may be too short-acting when used alone for most VR procedures. Therefore, 0.75% levobupivacaine with its longer duration of action is commonly used either in a 50:50 mixture with 2% lidocaine or as a single agent. Ropivacaine 0.75% is also suitable for use in VR surgery. Hyaluronidase is usually added to improve the onset and quality of the block.

Attainment of complete akinesia is a good indicator of the depth and quality of the block and typical volumes of LA required are 8ml for sub-Tenon's anaesthesia and 10ml for peribulbar block. With this approach, good, prolonged analgesia for surgery is readily achievable.

If greater depth of anaesthesia is needed during surgery, a sub-Tenon's injection on the table can be used to top up the initial block. It is not acceptable for surgery to proceed with the patient in pain and this may also make surgery more difficult and result in intraoperative patient movement and postoperative patient complaints.

Regional anaesthesia techniques after previous VR surgery

VR surgical procedures may result in difficulties with subsequent LA blocks.
- Sub-Tenon's block: medial port insertion sites for previous vitrectomy surgery may result in scarring such that it is difficult to discern the Tenon's capsule and to enter the medial sub-Tenon's space. There is also a risk of globe perforation if care is not taken when dissecting the scar tissue with scissors. Previous scleral buckle surgery may result in adhesions of Tenon's capsule (fascia) necessitating extra dissection of the Tenon's capsule to allow the passage of the sub-Tenon's cannula. The flow of LA around the globe is also affected and may result in an inadequate block

- Needle block: placement of an explant during scleral buckle surgery leads to distortion of the spherical nature of the globe's anatomy. This may increase the risk of globe perforation using a sharp needle technique

Biometry measurements

Biometry measurements of axial length are not usually available in VR surgery although axial myopia is a recognized risk factor for globe perforation during traditional needle blocks. However, studies in myopic eyes have shown that as the axial length of the eye increases, the increase in equatorial horizontal width was minimal. In addition, staphylomas are mainly located at the posterior pole of the globe with none at the equator. Therefore, if the single medial peribulbar approach is used, and the needle is directed backwards parallel to the medial orbital wall, the risk of ocular injuries is minimal. Sub-Tenon's or medial peribulbar anaesthesia is a safe technique in these eyes.

Role of sedation during regional anaesthesia

Sedation requirements vary by patient population and surgeon and anaesthetist preferences (see 📖 Aims of monitored sedation, p. 136). Some patients may require sedation to be able to tolerate VR surgery under RA. This may apply particularly to younger patients and those having scleral buckling procedures. Minimal sedation (anxiolysis) is preferable to deeper levels of sedation in order to prevent unpredictable movements. Midazolam is commonly used; other suitable drugs include propofol and remifentanil (see 📖 Drugs, p. 143).

Ensuring patient comfort and tolerance

The comfort of the patient makes a great difference in their ability to tolerate a long procedure under MAC and RA. Careful patient positioning on the operating table prior to the start of surgery is essential. Bony areas should be padded and a pillow placed under the knees to help relieve strain on the knees, hips and spine. Some centres allow patients a 'wriggle break' to adjust their positions every 30min or so to restore comfort. Ensuring an empty bladder prior to surgery is also sensible. If patients experience pain or discomfort during the procedure, the surgeon can readily supplement anaesthesia with a sub-Tenon's injection. Patients need to be informed of the procedure by which they alert the theatre team about any discomfort.

General anaesthesia

General anaesthesia

Although RA techniques are increasingly preferred for VR surgery there still remain some clear indications for GA.

Indications for GA in VR patients:

- Patient or surgeon preference
- Lengthy surgery—patients are often able to tolerate surgery of an hour in length but GA may be preferable for surgery of greater duration
- Patient factors such as movement disorders, claustrophobia, intractable cough
- Patient positioning problems
- Bilateral eye operations
- Communication difficulties such as deafness, dementia or language differences
- Absolute contraindications to LA including orbital infection and true allergy to LAs
- Relative contraindications such as only eye surgery and previous surgery in the same eye

Optimal operating conditions and goals of anaesthesia

The aims of GA for VR surgery are to ensure:

- Globe anaesthesia
- Globe and lid akinesia
- Normal or reduced IOP
- Avoidance of the oculo-cardiac reflex
- Avoidance of coughing on emergence
- Avoidance of postoperative nausea and vomiting

Practical implications

- The surgeon will require a well-anaesthetized eye remaining still in the neutral gaze position. Any gross sudden unexpected patient movement may result in injury to the eye that could lead to poor visual outcome. Depth of GA should be assured, otherwise a GA technique that includes muscle relaxation with mechanical ventilation should be considered. Neuromuscular transmission needs to be monitored to identify wearing off of relaxation and hence the risk of patient movement. A remifentanil infusion is helpful in addition to reduce respiratory drive and increase tolerance of either an endotracheal tube (ETT) or LMA
- Intra-ocular pressure can be reduced by mechanical ventilatory control of arterial carbon dioxide tension, avoiding tight ties around the neck and head-up positioning. Propofol and most intravenous anaesthetic agents reduce IOP
- Oculo-cardiac reflex (see 📖 Oculo-cardiac reflex, p. 44): the incidence of this reflex is high in VR surgery, especially procedures such as cryo-buckling surgery where traction on the extra-ocular muscles may precipitate it. The reflex involves branches of the trigeminal nerve in the afferent limb and the vagus nerve in the efferent limb. Stimulation can result in severe bradycardia or cardiac standstill and may be a factor in the high incidence of postoperative nausea and vomiting. The afferent limb can be attenuated by using a LA block in addition to GA

and this has been shown to reduce its incidence. The efferent limb is blocked by anticholinergic agents such as glycopyrrolate.

- Airway management. Access to the airway is limited during VR surgery and it is essential that the airway is secured. The use of a reinforced or flexible supraglottic airway is a very satisfactory way of managing the airway. It avoids laryngoscopy which can result in hypertension and increased IOP. Its presence is less stimulating than that of an endotracheal tube so there is reduced likelihood of intraoperative movement or coughing on emergence. If an ETT is used then smoother emergence can be achieved by lidocaine spray to the cords, intravenous lidocaine, remifentanil infusion, and other techniques.

- Postoperative nausea and vomiting (PONV) is common after general anaesthesia (see 📖 Postoperative nausea and vomiting, p. 378) for VR surgery. Vomiting can result in a sudden rise in IOP with the potential to cause serious eye complications including intra-ocular haemorrhage, wound rupture, loss of vitreous. and iris prolapse. In those patients who have received intra-ocular gas injection, vomiting may also interfere with postoperative posturing. The use of intraoperative antiemetics reduces the incidence of PONV; combinations of $5HT_3$ antagonists, dexamethasone, and cyclizine are popular in eye surgery. Propofol is antiemetic and PONV is reduced by total intravenous anaesthesia (TIVA) with propofol. Avoidance of nitrous oxide may also be beneficial. LA block in addition to general anaesthesia has been shown to reduce PONV possibly due to the attenuation of the oculo-emetic reflex and through the decreased requirement for opioids.

General anaesthetic technique

- An example technique of GA for VR surgery is as follows:
  - Intravenous induction with propofol
  - Relaxation with non-depolarizing muscle relaxant
  - Reinforced supraglottic airway unless contraindicated
  - Maintenance: TIVA with propofol and remifentanil. Intermittent positive pressure ventilation. Monitoring of neuromuscular blockade
  - Additional LA block
  - Use of antiemetics

Monitoring

Careful patient monitoring with appropriate alarms is essential during VR surgery under both LA and GA. This is because of the darkened theatre environment, the age and associated medical conditions of many of these patients, and the risk of precipitating cardiac arrhythmias from drugs used (such as mydricaine) and the oculo-cardiac reflex.

Nitrous oxide

In some VR procedures, intra-ocular gases are used to tamponade the retina. If nitrous oxide is used as part of an anaesthetic it can diffuse into this gas bubble causing it to expand and so lead to a rise in IOP. Increases in IOP above the perfusion pressure of the central artery of the retina may occlude this artery and so result in permanent blindness.

Nitrous oxide can be used during VR surgery as the diffusion of nitrous oxide into intra-ocular gas bubbles is time-dependent and if gas is introduced just before the end of surgery, then the effects of nitrous oxide would be negligible. A problem arises when surgery on the first eye has finished and an additional procedure is performed on the other eye. Then, nitrous oxide should be avoided or turned off as soon as the first eye has been closed.

Patients with pre-existing gas bubbles who have a subsequent GA with nitrous oxide are at particular risk. There have been several case reports of irreversible blindness following nitrous oxide anaesthesia in the presence of an intra-ocular gas bubble. Perfluoropropane gas (C_3F_8) is particularly long-acting and the risk with nitrous oxide anaesthesia may remain for several weeks.

Patients must be warned of the risks and should be provided with a notification bracelet to alert future anaesthetists.

Mydricaine

Mydricaine is used in some VR units to ensure a fully dilated pupil of long duration. It is injected into the subconjunctival space and contains procaine, atropine, and adrenaline. It has been known to cause adverse cardiovascular effects such as severe hypertension, cardiac arrhythmias, and myocardial infarction. Tachycardia and transient myocardial ischaemia have been reported in patients with no previous history of ischaemic heart disease and can occur even with lower concentrations of solution. If mydricaine is used then the surgeon must warn the anaesthetist and the patient must be closely monitored.

Lasers in VR surgery

Laser treatment is often used during VR surgery and the usual precautions when using lasers in theatre must be adhered.

Postoperative care

Postoperative postures

Following VR surgery patients may need to adopt a particular posture to ensure that the gas bubble in the eye is in the optimal position. When the retinal break is superior, the optimal position is sitting upright and if the hole is posterior the optimal position is face down. Patients are able to posture immediately after surgery if RA and MAC has been used. If GA is used then the patient will have to recover sufficiently before they are able to adopt the optimal position.

Pain relief

Mild to moderate pain is common after VR surgery. This is effectively treated with combinations of simple analgesics such as paracetamol and NSAIDs (see ▢ Postoperative pain management, pp. 376–377). Morphine is rarely required and has unwanted effects of causing nausea and vomiting and excessive sedation. The use of RA either as a sole technique or in combination with GA greatly reduces postoperative pain especially if a long-acting agent is used and is recommended.

Conclusion

VR surgery is performed both under general and increasingly under regional ophthalmic anaesthesia. The requirement of anaesthesia varies and the duration of surgical procedure is unpredictable, hence necessary precautions must be taken.

Key reading

Keay L, Lindsley K, Tielsch J, Katz J, Schein O. *Routine preoperative medical testing for cataract surgery (review)*. The Cochrane Collaboration, 2009.

The Royal College of Anaesthetists and The Royal College of Ophthalmologists. *Local anaesthesia for intraocular surgery*. 2001; London: The Royal College of Anaesthetists and The Royal College of Ophthalmologists.

Chapter 16

Anaesthesia for adult strabismus surgery

Dr Shashi Vohra

Introduction

Adult patients present for strabismus surgery for a primary correction, or for revision of previously failed surgery. Strabismus is either congenital or acquired. It is generally caused by paralysis of extra-ocular muscles resulting from damage to the IIIrd, IVth or VIth cranial nerves or it may be due to the inherent weakness of the muscles themselves. Other causes include endocrinal disorders such as dysthyroid disease leading to mechanical restriction, fibrosis, entrapment or overactivity of the extra-ocular muscles. Diabetes causes strabismus via intracranial microvascular pathology. Occasionally patients may present for correction of their visual axis following macular rotation or scleral buckling for retinal detachment.

- Surgery may be unilateral or bilateral and involve one or two muscles in each eye
- Surgery is aimed at:
  - Weakening the strong muscle by resection or myectomy
  - Strengthening the weak muscle by muscle tuck or advancement
- Key anaesthesia concerns include:
  - Associated comorbidities
  - Ocular-cardiac reflex (OCR)
  - Oculocemetric reflex
  - Potential malignant hyperthermia
  - Postoperative nausea and vomiting (PONV)

Syndromes associated with strabismus

There are several syndromes that are associated with congenital or acquired strabismus. Syndromic patients may pose a variety of anaesthetic challenges. This list of syndromes is not exhaustive.

- Down's syndrome: 20% may have strabismus. Patients typically exhibit microgenia, macroglossia, cervical spine abnormalities, decreased muscle tone, cardiac abnormalities and are at high risk for gastro-oesophageal reflux, obstructive sleep apnoea, and sensitivity to anaesthetic drugs
- Mobius syndrome: failure of eye abduction, skeletal abnormalities, and palatal weakness
- Ehlers–Danlos syndromes: hypermobile joints, kyphoscoliosis, and diaphragmatic hernia
- Whistling face or Freeman–Sheldon syndrome: increased muscle tone, very small mouth

Intracranial pathology

Patients often have associated neurological or endocrinal deficit depending on the extent of the causative lesion:

- Oculomotor nerve palsy (IIIrd cranial nerve) is associated with cerebellar ataxia in Nothangel's syndrome
  - Hemitremor (Benedict's syndrome)
  - Contralateral hemiparesis (Weber's syndrome)
- Abducens nerve palsy (VIth cranial nerve) may be associated with:
  - Intracranial haemorrhage
  - Infection
  - Infiltration
  - Carcinoma involving brainstem, subarachnoid space, petrous temporal bone, cavernous sinus or orbit
- Trochlear (IVth cranial nerve) palsy is caused by neoplasms in 10% of cases, 20% are ischaemic, 30% are due to miscellaneous causes and 40% result from trauma

The description of various syndromes is beyond the scope of this chapter and the reader is referred to neuro-opthalmology or paedaitric anaesthesia textbooks.

History and physical examination

History should include general enquiries relevant to the conduct of GA as well as questions specific to conditions associated with strabismus.

- Past medical history therefore should include questions about:
  - Birth hypoxia
  - Head injury
  - Epilepsy
  - Cerebrovascular accident (CVA)
  - Intracranial tumours prior surgery
- Syndromic patients may have:
  - Mental retardation
  - Muscle weakness
  - Airway problems
  - Skeletal disorders
  - Metabolic and cardiac abnormalities
- Family history should include questions about:
  - Myopathies
  - Malignant hyperpyrexia
  - Epilepsy and any drug reactions
- Examination should focus on:
  - Routine enquiries
  - Evidence of comorbidities particularly other neuromuscular disorders or unrecognized cardiomiopathy
  - Syndromic features
  - History of postoperative retching, nausea, vomiting
  - History of motion sickness
  - Familial presence of muscle disease
  - Familial history of malignant hyperthermia or unexplained untoward reactions to general anaesthetics

General and systemic examination

Routine general examination: height, weight, body mass index (BMI) etc.

- Syndromic features
- Cardiovascular system: heart rate, blood pressure, heart sounds, and murmurs
- Respiratory system: clubbing, respiratory rate, chest expansion, tracheal position, tracheotomy scars etc.:
  - Some patients may have had tracheotosmy following head injury or intracranial surgery
  - Previous thyroid surgery may also have residual airway involvement
- Musculoskeletal: range of neck movement, jaw, dentition, tremor, abnormal movements, and mobility

Investigations

- Routine laboratory tests are not recommended

General anaesthesia

Premedication

- Premedication aims to allay anxiety and to prevent PONV
- Prophylactic treatment with anticholinergic drugs is controversial and generally not recommended:
  - Timing of intramuscular injections such that maximal effectiveness is achieved at the time of surgical stimulus and potential OCR is difficult
  - Intravenous anticholinergic may be administered at the time of IV placement or immediately prior to the start of surgical stimulus

Induction

- Surgery typically takes between 25–30min per muscle and may last for over an hour with bilateral surgery
- Choice of drugs depends on whether ventilation is to be controlled or not
- Induction of anaesthesia may be accomplished with any suitable induction agent. Propofol has an added advantage of quick recovery profile particularly for day cases. It also possesses antiemetic properties
- Those not suitable for propofol (e.g. allergy to its components), thiopentone or etomidate may be used
- Midazolam as a co-induction drug reduces the dose of induction agent and provides amnesia
- Analgesia is provided by fentanyl, alfentanil or a remifentanil infusion
- Airway may be secured with a reinforced LMA if there are no specific contraindications such as uncontrolled gastrooesophageal reflux
- Many clinicians prefer to use an endotracheal tube, e.g. Rae or a re-inforced tube. Others prefer supraglottic airways (LMA).
- It is important that airway is secured properly and remains accessible under the drapes
- Non-depolarizing relaxant such as vecuronium, rocuronium, mivacurium or atracurium is used to facilitate muscle relaxation and IPPV

Maintenance

- Anaesthesia is maintained with an inhalation agent such as isoflurane, sevoflurane, or desflurane in a mixture of nitrous oxide and oxygen or air
- Alternatively, infusion of target-controlled propofol and remifentanil infusion may be used if facilities exist
- Ventilation may be spontaneous, augmented or controlled
- Analgesia is maintained with opiates such as fentanyl/remifentanil and may be supplemented with intravenous paracetamol or NSAIDs

Monitoring

Standard monitoring such as ECG, pulse oximeter, non-invasive blood pressure, inhalation agent, inspired gases, $EtCO_2$ and temperature should be used. Additional monitoring is dictated by patient-specific comorbidities and intraoperative events.

Intraoperative considerations

Oculo-cardiac reflex (OCR)

OCR is generally elicited by traction on extra-ocular muscles and/or pressure and manipulation of the globe or orbit. All extra-ocular muscles have been implicated (see 📖 Extra-ocular muscles, pp. 26–28).

- Predisposing factors include hypoxia, hypercarbia, and light planes of anaesthesia
- Neuromuscular block of the extra-ocular muscles with peripheral neuromuscular blocking agents does not prevent OCR
- The OCR usual manifests as bradycardia, supraventricular ectopy, junctional rhythm, and atriventricular conduction blocks
- More serious disturbance may include ventricular bigeminy and multifocal ventricular ectopics
- Transient asystole is not uncommon
- The afferent arc of the OCR is through the ophthalmic branch of the trigeminal nerve. The impulses are conveyed via long and short ciliary nerves to the gassesrian ganglion (Vth cranial nerve). The central connections are at midbrain level with the Xth cranial nerve (vagus) nucleus. The efferent pathway is via the cardio-inhibitory fibres of the vagus nerve
- As the reflex displays tachyphylaxis, repeated stimuli are often accompanied by attenuated responses
- First action should be cessation of the surgical stimulus by release of extra-ocular muscle traction or pressure on the globe. Allow the heart rate and rhythm to return to baseline while simultaneously ensuring adequate oxygenation ventilation and depth of anaesthesia
- Minor haemodynamic instability of brief duration may not require the use of anticholinergics
- Major haemodynamic instability warrants urgent use of atropine or glycopyrrolate, atropine is the appropriate first agent for urgently mediated symptomatic bradysrhythmia. Caution is required in elderly patients, especially those with ischaemic heart disease, as prolonged tachycardia resulting from a full vagolytic dose may precipitate ischaemia
- The OCR may be prevented by interrupting the afferent limb of the arc by use of regional ophthalmic block. The use of short-acting LA is recommended if postoperative adjustment of sutures is planned as residual anaesthetic effect can result in poor alignment

Oculo-respiratory reflex

- In spontaneously breathing patients the oculo-respiratory reflex is manifested as irregular shallow breathing culminating in apnoea. The afferent impulses are carried via long and short ciliary nerves to the sensory nucleus of the trigeminal nerve and the efferent pathway is via the respiratory centres of pons and medulla

Oculo-emetic reflex

- This reflex is implicated, although not proven, for causing PONV. A central imbalance caused by the disparity between the visual and vestibular impulses during postoperative mobilization is a suggested hypothesis for its causation

Forced duction test

- The forced duction test (FDT) is used to differentiate between a mechanical and the paralytic aetiology of the strabismus
- Globe movement is tested by applying a traction on the relevant muscle. Full range of movement is expected
- This test is said to be positive when mechanical tethering resulting from previous scarring or endocrinal orbitopathy prevents full range of globe movement
- The eye muscles need to be fully relaxed as persistent residual tone due to inadequate relaxation leads to misinterpretation of the test. A survey has found that 55% of paediatric and 66% of adult patients had residual muscle tone during forced duction test and therefore may have had surgery under suboptimal surgical conditions. Suxamethonium may render the forced duction test unreliable because extra-ocular muscles have preponderance of neuromuscular junctions. Repeated firing after suxamethonium results in contracture of the muscles and abnormal tone which may persist for up to 20min. Therefore, the use of a non-depolarizing muscle relaxant should be considered if FDT is to be employed

Strabismus and malignant hyperthermia

Suxamethonium is generally not advocated in patients presenting for strabismus surgery. A link between malignant hyperpyrexia, inherited myopathies, and strabismus surgery has been observed particularly in paediatric patients. A thorough history of previous exposure to triggering agents and any complications should be explored.

Regional anaesthesia for strabismus surgery

Regional anaesthesia (RA) such as extraconal (peribulbar), intraconal (retrobulbar) or sub-Tenon's blocks is also used for adult strabismus surgery.

- RA usually blocks the afferent limb of the OCR, however, note that it may initially trigger the reflex prior to onset of anaesthesia
- RA is associated with a lower incidence of PONV
- RA is generally reserved for unilateral surgery but carefully conducted and timed 'staggered' blocks for bilateral surgery in the same sitting have been described:
  - The first block is performed by the anaesthetist or surgeon and both eyes are prepared and draped. Following completion of the first eye surgery, the second block is done by the surgeon without disturbing the surgical field and asepsis
  - Staggering the blocks mitigates the potential local and systemic complications of simultaneous bilateral injections
- Topical anaesthesia or deep fornix block, although not commonly practiced, may have a role in selected patients. Topical 2% lignocaine gel has been shown to provide better analgesia than 1% amethocaine. Topical anaesthesia may be supplemented with subconjunctival infiltration to improve surgical conditions

Postoperative management

Nausea and vomiting

There is usually high incidence of PONV following strabismus surgery (see 📖 Postoperative nausea and vomiting, p. 378). An incidence of 30–40% has been quoted in the literature. Delayed oral intake may lead to dehydration, electrolyte imbalance, and unanticipated admission to an impatient facility.

Prevention is based on general principles:

- Preoperative anxiety is associated with PONV. Consider premedication with a benzodiazepine
- Propofol has antiemetic properties but is associated with a higher incidence of intraoperative bradycardia and OCR
- Use of TIVA
- Avoidance of opiates
- Nitrous oxide-free anaesthesia (debatable)
- Avoidance of long-acting neuromuscular blockers that may require proemetic anticholiaesterase reversal
- LMA obviates the need for neuromuscular blockade and subsequent use of anticholiaesterase reversal
- Intraoperative prophylactic usage of $5HT_3$ receptor blockers such as intravenous ondansetron (4–8mg; 100mic/Kg) alone or in combination with other antiemetics. Combination therapy is more effective than individual drugs
- Droperidol has been the most widely studied and considered the gold standard antiemetic for strabismus surgery patients, however there may be some concerns with prolongation of the QT interval
- Adequate hydration
- Gentle surgical handling of the eye muscles
- Ophthalmic regional block prior to emergence from anaesthesia decreases the incidence of PONV
- Non-pharmacologic manoeuvres such as use of an acupressure device
- Avoid premature inducement to eat

Analgesia

Oral or intramuscular codeine with or without paracetamol is usually adequate as the surgery evokes only moderate pain. Non-steroidal analgesics although a useful adjunct have the theoretical disadvantage of platelet inhibition in susceptible individuals which may interfere with the delicate surgical procedure besides causing gastrointestinal irritation. LA such as sub-Tenon's block intraoperatively or towards the end of the surgical procedure is sometimes used to obtain postoperative pain relief. However, this mode of analgesia is undesirable if the procedure involves adjustment of suture in the postoperative period.

Postoperative adjustment of sutures

Adjustment of sutures is carried out to fine-tune the surgical correction and balance the visual axes. The procedure is done in the postoperative period following recovery from anaesthesia. It requires patients to be fully awake and cooperative otherwise there is a risk of under- or overcorrection. The timing between recovery and the adjustment depends on surgeon's preference and the type of anaesthetic used for the main surgical procedure.

- Topical local anaesthetic eye drops are used to provide analgesia
- Some surgeons may use topical vasoconstrictors to provide ischaemic field and prevent conjunctival and episcleral haemorrhage. Dilute epinephrine is traditionally used. It may however have adverse haemodynamic effect in addition to causing mydriasis which interferes with accommodation needed for adjustment of sutures
- Alternatives such as topical α2-adrenergic agonists (0.2% brimonidine 0.2% and 1% apraclonidine 1%) have been described in selected patients
- Patients may experience fainting, dizziness, nausea, and vomiting during adjustment of sutures due to vasovagal or OCR described earlier

It is advisable to monitor vital signs during adjustment of sutures and have resuscitative facilities available.

Conclusion

Strabismus surgery realigns the visual axes. Anaesthesia for most adult patients is conducted via block and sedation. GA is employed for paediatric patients. These include patients with congenital or acquired syndromes and those in whom the aetiology is associated with neurological, metabolic or endocrine factors. The aim of the anaesthetic management is to identify, quantify and manage the individual risk factors and plan the anaesthetic accordingly.

Key reading

Brown DR, Pacheco EM, Repka MX. Recovery of extraocular muscle function after adjustable suture strabismus surgery under local anesthesia. *J. Pediatr. Opthalmol. Strabismus.* 1992; 29(1): 16–20.

Dahlmann-Noor AH, Cosgrave E, Lowe S, Bailly M, Vivian JA. Brimonidine and apraclonidine as vasoconstrictors in adjustable strabismus surgery. *J. of AAPOS.* 2009; 13(2): 123–6.

Dell R, Williams B. Anaesthesia for strabismus surgery: a regional survey. *Br. J. Anaesth.* 1999; 82(5): 761–3.

Chapter 17

Anaesthesia for adult corneal transplant surgery

Dr Shashi Vohra

Introduction

Corneal transplant/graft surgery involves removal of damaged host cornea and its replacement with a healthy cornea from the eye of a suitable donor.

- The indications for corneal transplant generally include:
  - Correction of corneal deformity
  - Treatment of intractable pain
  - Unresponsive infection
- Transplants are classified as:
  - Optical
  - Tectonic
  - Therapeutic
  - Cosmetic
- The specific indications are:
  - Keratoconus
  - Keratoglobus
  - Fuchs' endothelial dystrophy
  - Pseudophakic bullous keratopathy
  - Corneal scars or opacity resulting from trauma, chemicals, perforation or infection
- Demographics:
  - All age groups
  - Elderly with comorbidities during anaesthesia

Transplant terminology

Penetrating keratoplasty

This procedure involves a full-thickness graft of the cornea with a donor's tissue.

- This is an 'open roof' or 'open sky' technique
- The host cornea is excised with a trephine. A full-thickness donor corneal scleral button is fashioned with a trephine from donor corneal scleral tissue to suit the host and sutured in place. The donor tissue is screened for potential infective organisms such as hepatitis, human immunodeficiency virus (HIV), syphilis etc., and examined for optical quality
- Tissue typing is usually not necessary

Anterior lamellar keratoplasty

- For patients with diseases affecting the anterior part of the cornea. These include keratoconus, corneal dystrophy, and scarring resulting from herpes infection
- In some dystrophies only the anterior half of the corneal stroma is removed, whereas in others (keratoconus), almost the entire anterior corneal stroma is dissected away from the posterior lamellar leaving the Descemet's membrane and endothelium
- The dissected anterior tissue is replaced by donor tissue with the endothelium, Descemet's membrane and occasionally lamellar of the posterior stroma are removed
- The incidence of rejection is generally lower and the potential complications of a full-thickness graft are avoided

Descemet's stripping endothelial keratoplasty (DSEK)

This relatively new procedure is indicated in patients with decompensated corneal endothelium.

- The surgical indications include Fuch's dystrophy, trauma, and bullous keratopathy
- These patients tend to develop corneal oedema because they are unable to maintain corneal deturgescence and corneal clarity
- The surgical process involves using a very thin donor endothelial layer supported by the adjacent Descemet's membrane for transplant
- The diseased corneal endothelium is gently dissected from the internal (posterior) surface of the recipient cornea through a small limbal incision
- An automated keratome is used to procure a <50 micron thick posterior lamellar from the donor cornea compromising mainly the endothelial monolayer Descemet's membrane
- This tissue is then floated into the anterior chamber of the eye through the small peripheral limbal opening
- The graft is drawn in, tamponaded with air and is 'held' in place by donor endothelial electrostatic forces at the graft–host interface

Epikeratophakia

For patients with pathologically thinned cornea (keratoconus or keratoglobus):

- The technique involves suturing of a large donor lamellar corneal disc or commercially available corneal lenticule, over a de-epithelialized host cornea
- A modified technique involves a *two-stage* process:
  - The first stage is a closed eye procedure to strengthen a thin scarred eye. This requires removal of the donor corneal endothelium from a large cornea-scleral rim which is then sutured as an overlay onto the recipient's de-epithelialized ocular surface
  - The second stage is an 'open roof' procedure involving a full-thickness penetrating keratoplasty as described above

Tectonic keratoplasty

Patients suffering from severe autoimmune disorders such as rheumatoid arthritis, Wegener's granulomatosis, Stevens–Johnson syndrome, toxic epidermal necrolysis, mucous membrane pemphigoid, or severe microbial keratitis may develop spontaneous destructive corneal perforations which cannot be closed with glue or amniotic membrane tissue grafting.

- Ongoing inflammatory processes with severe recurrent corneal melts are rare. In these cases urgent tectonic keratoplasty is indicated
- May take the form of either a lamellar or full thickness penetrating transplant
- Patients tend to be frail with a host of other comorbidities, making them a high risk for general anaesthesia

Phototherapeutic keratectomy

For patients with diseased, friable corneal epithelium (recurrent corneal erosion syndrome) resulting from diabetes, fingernail trauma, and some hereditary corneal dystrophies.

- The irregular damaged epithelial surface of the host cornea is removed
- The Bowman's layer of the donor cornea is ablated to a depth of ~7.5–10mcg by an excimer laser and grafted on to the prepared external host corneal surface
- The release of tissue-specific inflammatory mediators and growth factors facilitates adhesion of the migrating host epithelium to the underlying basement membrane/Bowman's layer of the donor cornea

Anaesthetic implications and choice of anaesthesia technique

Penetrating keratoplasty 'open roof' procedures carry a high risk of expulsion of globe contents and expulsive suprachoroidal haemorrhage.

- In non-penetrating keratoplasties, a combination of other procedures such as extracapsular cataract extraction, anterior segment reconstruction or vitrectomy renders them equally hazardous as an open procedure
- Anaesthesia considerations include:
  - Maintenance of normal IOP and prevention of fluctuations
  - Prevention of eye squeezing
  - Avoidance of intraoperative cough and movement
  - Extra-ocular muscle relaxation
  - Maintenance of retinal vein and artery perfusion
  - Position of the anaesthetist remote from the patient's airway assuring there is no gross movement during critical portions of the procedure. For regional anaesthesia this is primarily patient-dependent but for general anaesthesia it is anaesthetist-dependent

Choice of anaesthetic technique

The choice of the anaesthetic technique depends on the surgical procedure, anaesthetist's and surgeon's preferences and experience as well as the clinical condition of the patient.

- There is wide variation in preferred anaesthesia techniques
- General anaesthesia:
  - No surgical time constraint
  - Avoids the anxiety around the patient's ability to stay still for the duration of surgery
  - Secure airway
- Regional anaesthesia with MAC
  - Ideal for patients who are at risk for general anaesthesia such as the older elderly and those with a difficult airway (several rheumatoid arthritis):
  - Patient maintains airway
  - Patient must be able to remain relatively still for the duration of surgery
  - Limited utility for procedures greater than 2h duration
  - Tissue scarring may inhibit spread of LA, resulting in less satisfactory results
- Topical anaesthesia:
  - Limited utility

General anaesthesia

Preoperative assessment

- History, examination and investigations:
  - Past and current medical history should include routine questions as well as enquiries as to the aetiology of the eye injury
  - Drug history is important as concurrent medication has implications on the conduct of anaesthesia and drug interactions
  - Immunosuppressants such as cyclosporine or methotrexate may result in bone marrow suppression
  - Patients may be on steroids or anticoagulant or antiplatelet drugs such as warfarin, clopidogrel or aspirin. The decision to discontinue these would rest with haematologist or cardiologist, patient's condition, and the surgical preference
  - Patients with Stevens–Johnson syndrome may have sensitivity to anaesthetic agents, most commonly NSAIDs
  - Routine and specific haematological, biochemical or cardiac investigations are dictated by age and the comorbidities of the individual patient

Premedication

- In adult patients this may include anxiolytics (e.g. benzodiazepines such as oral temazepam), antiemetics/prokinetics (metoclopramide) and histamine receptor (H_2) blockers (ranitidine) where indicated
- Pediatric patients may benefit from oral benzodinepines
- Premedication with anxiolytics can allay separation anxiety for both the child and the parents

Induction and maintenance

- As with eye procedures in general, fluctuations in intra-ocular pressure should be minimized
- Induction of anaesthesia should be smooth
- General anaesthesia may be induced with any suitable intravenous agent (propofol, thiopentone or etomidate)
- Ketamine is controversial. It may carry a risk of increasing IOP
- Midazolam may be used as a co-induction agent
- Analgesia is provided with fentanyl or alternatively remifentanil infusion which may be continued intraoperatively. NSAIDs may be contradicted for patients with history of Stevens–Johnson syndrome.
- Traditionally, the airway is secured with an endotracheal tube:
  - Direct laryngoscopy and intubation raises IOP
  - Increased risk of bucking or coughing during maintenance phase and emergence from GA
- Supraglottic airway may be preferable:
  - Minimal/no effect on IOP during induction, maintenance, and emergence from GA
  - Proper fit must be assured prior to onset of surgery as adjustment intraoperatively may be difficult
- Airway should be secure and accessible under the drapes

- Adequate depth of anaesthesia, muscle relaxation, and normocarbia must be maintained throughout the surgery
- Coughing or bucking must be diligently avoided
- IOP should be maintained at normal levels by taking general and preventive measures. Specific measures may include:
  - Intravenous acetazolamide
  - Mannitol
  - Lidocaine should be readily available to attempt to minimize any sudden increase in IOP
  - Avoid rise in venous congestion by careful positioning of the head and neck and maintaining slight reverse Trendelenberg position
- Autonomic stability should be maintained to avoid sudden surges in systemic blood pressure which may carry a risk of suprachoroidal haemorrhage
- Suprachoroidal haemorrhage (SCH) is a rare but most dreaded complication of intra-ocular surgery. It manifests as a sudden haemorrhage in the choroid during surgery resulting in expulsion of contents of the globe and immediate loss of vision
- SCH may occur spontaneously. It is an exceedingly rare occurrence with cataract or transplant surgery
- Predisposing factors for SCH:
  - Atherosclerotic peripheral vascular disease
  - Uncontrolled chronic systemic
  - Ocular hypertension
  - Sudden changes in the IOP
  - Congenital or acquired coagulopathies
  - Systemic anticoagulants
  - Antiplatelet agents
  - Diabetes
  - Inflammatory ocular disease
  - Previous surgery
- Even with prompt treatment, the outcome may not be favourable

Regional anaesthesia

Regional anaesthesia (orbital block) may be considered for select procedures and patients, depending on the procedure and patient, surgeon and anaesthetist's preferences and experience.

- Keratoplasties retrobulbar, peribulbar) as well as blunt cannula-based block (sub-Tenon's block).
- Hyaluronidase may be used to speed the onset of the block, to enhance spread of LA, and to reduce fluctuations in the IOP.
- Use of an oculocompression device depends on ocular pathology and surgeon/anaesthetist preference.
- Patients presenting with gross infection, glaucoma, bullous keratopathy, and graft rejection may not be suitable for RA.
  - Photophobia, redness, blurred vision, blepharospasm, and pain may make RA technically difficult.
  - Insertion of eye speculum during sub-Tenon's block may be painful
  - Hyperaemic conjunctiva increases the risk of subconjunctival haemorrhage
  - Supplemental topical anaesthetic drops and choosing an avascular area of conjunctiva may help reduce discomfort and prevent the haemorrhage
- Non-akinetic anaesthesia techniques such as topical anaesthesia combined with intra-cameral supplementation of LA have also been described for select patients:
  - Reserved for those rare patients with marked risk from GA and RA
  - Topical anaesthetic drops may be supplemented with subconjuctival limbal injections of LA

Monitored anaesthesia care

- Intraoperatively patient should be made comfortable by supporting bony points (hips, knees and elbows)
- Warming blanket may be required for longer procedures
- The surgical drape should be tented near the patient's face to prevent hypercarbia and a suction tube positioned near patient's head may be helpful
- Fresh gas (oxygen/air) should be supplied under the drapes
- Explicit instructions must be given to patients to remain relatively still and avoid sudden movements. In the event the movement becomes unavoidable they should be instructed to warn the operating team prior to moving
- A slight head-up position may help reduce the risks of raised venous congestion and IOP
- Care should be taken with the preoperative use of acetazolamide or mannitol as they may result in full bladder
- Obstructive uropathy if present in elderly male patients may lead to intraoperative restlessness and sudden movements
- Use of oral preoperative codeine as an antitussive agent to control cough may be useful, although the patient and surgeon must understand that it is not a guarantee of full intraoperative cough suppression
- Lidocaine should be readily available to mitigate a sudden elevation of IOP
- Loss of verbal contact in the dark environment of the operating room theatre may result in sleep/awake cycle leading to sudden movement of the head which can jeopardise surgical outcome
- Respiratory depression and inadequate ventilation may also lead to nausea, restlessness, and confusion as well as haemodynamic disturbances
- Elderly patients may respond unpredictably to sedative drugs
- Sedation is no substitute to an inadequate block. The quality of the block should be judged carefully before commencing the surgery

Postoperative care

- Sudden, abrupt increases in IOP upon emergence from general anaesthesia may result in postoperative complications and poor ultimate visual outcome
- Emergence from anaesthesia should be smooth without undue coughing and retching
- Modern drugs such as remifentanil and sevoflurane/desflurane when used judiciously provide reliable and predictable course of anaesthesia
- Particular care should be taken to prevent PONV. Strategies that may minimize likelihood of PONV include:
  - Avoidance of gastric insufflation during induction/intubation
  - Adequate hydration
  - Maintenance of normothermia
  - Normoglycaemia
  - Avoidance of excessive oropharyngeal toilet
  - Avoidance of long acting opiates and nitrous oxide
  - Prophylactic use of combination therapy such as 5-HT$_3$ receptor blockers (e.g. ondansetron 4–8mg), antihistamines e.g. cyclizine (50mg) or benadryl (25–50mg) and dexamethasone (4–8mg)
- Postoperative analgesia can be provided with a combination of paracetamol, codeine and/or NSAIDs provided there are no specific contraindications
- Regional anaesthetic block prior to emergence for management of postoperative pain is advisable

Recent advances in corneal transplantation

Corneal limbal stem cell transplantation

- Limbal disease results in failure of regeneration of corneal epithelial cells
- Traditional corneal transplant is not suitable for pathology affecting the limbus as it only replaces the central part of the cornea. Involves dissection of damaged limbal tissue from the host corneal limbal stem, cell transplantation involves cornea
- Donor limbal stem cell tissue is obtained as an allograft from a deceased eye, a living related donor, or an autograft from the patient's contralateral healthy eye
- The donor tissue is then sutured on to the prepared host bed enabling repopulation of the corneal surface by donor epithelial cells

Synthetic cornea

Other new developments include use of synthetic corneas (keratoprostheses) for patients with recurrent graft failure, repeated rejection or those with highly vascularized cornea in whom the traditional cornea transplant would be ineffective.

Osteo-odonto-keratoprosthesis

- A multi-stage procedure that uses a patient's own tooth root and alveolar bone to support an optical lens. This keratoprosthetic complex is grafted to replace damaged cornea
- Suitable for patients for whom other techniques of corneal transplant are not appropriate, such as those with Stevens–Johnson syndrome or chemical injury
- GA is required for each staged procedure. History of drug allergy should be noted, particularly if the aetiology of corneal disease was due to Stevens–Johnson-type drug reaction. Procedures tend to be quite lengthy in duration, so particular attention to positioning and pressure points is indicated. Consider placement of a urinary catheter

Conclusion

Anaesthesia for corneal transplant surgery can be challenging due to the complex nature of the surgery. Patients may have significant comorbidities. Surgical techniques are constantly evolving. The intricacies of the surgical procedure and their anaesthetic implications need to be discussed with the patient and the surgeon prior to surgery. There are a number of options for specific anaesthesia techniques. Prescription of a suitable method is dependent on procedures, patient, surgeon, and anaesthesia-dependent factors.

Acknowledgement

The author wishes to thank Miss S Rauz, Consultant ophthalmologist, Birmingham Midland eye centre for her help with corneal transplant terminologies.

Key reading

Chu TG, Green RL. Suprachoroidal hemorrhage. *Surv. Ophthalmol.* 1999; 43: 471–86.

Garzozi HJ, Shehadeh-Masha'our R, Somri M, Kagemann L, Harris A. The effects of droperidol in perforating keratoplasty. *Ophthalmologica.* 2006; 220/4: 242–5.

Liu C, Okera S, Tandon R, Herold J, Hull C, Thorp S. Visual rehabilitation in end-stage inflammatory ocular surface disease with the osteo-odontokeratoprosthesis: results from the UK. *Br. J. Ophthalmol.* 2008; 92: 1211–17.

Muraine M, Calenda E, Watt L, Proust N et al. Peribulbar anaesthesia during keratoplasty: a prospective study of 100 cases. *Br J Ophthalmol.* 1999; 83: 104–9.

Rauz S, Saw VP. Serum eye drops, amniotic membrane and limbal epithelial stem cells—tools in the treatment of ocular surface disease. *Cell Tissue Bank.* 22 April 2009 DOI 10.1007/s10561-009-9128-1.

Segev F, Voineaskos F, Hui G, Law MS, Paul R et al. Combined topical and intracameral anesthesia in penetrating keratoplasty. *Cornea.* 2004; 23(4): 372–6.

Anaesthesia for tumour surgery

Professor Steven Gayer

Introduction

Ocular cancer is classified based upon histology, anatomic location, and the extent of growth. Orbital tumours may be:
- Primary or secondary
- Benign or malignant
- Intra-ocular, extra-ocular or intra-ocular with extra-ocular extension

Secondary tumours may result from metastatic spread from distant locations or very rarely as a direct extension of an extra-ocular tumour into the eye.

Primary histotypes include:
- Melanoma
- Retinoblastoma
- Lymphoma
- Haemangioma
- Astrocytoma

Melanoma and retinoblastoma have the most significant anaesthetic implications and will be the focus of this chapter.

Anatomical considerations

The globe's posterior portion is comprised of three layers:
- The sclera is a tough, avascular outer layer that provides rigidity and structural support
- The uveal tract is the highly vascular middle layer
- The inner retina which contains the neural photoreceptor network
The uveal tract is comprised of three layers:
  - The choroid which provides a vascular conduit for the retina
  - The ciliary body is the anterior extension of the choroid. It produces aqueous humour which contributes to maintaining intra-ocular pressure. It also makes accommodation possible by using its internal musculature to alter the shape of the lens
  - The iris, which is continuous with the ciliary body, consists of a ring of pigmented tissue surrounding the pupil. It serves to regulate the amount of light allowed into the eye

Location

Primary ocular tumours may be found throughout the eye, including:
- Choroid:
  - Choroidal melanoma
  - Choroidal metastases
  - Choroidal naevus
  - Choroidal haemangioma
- Ciliary body:
  - Ciliary body melanoma
  - Epithelioma
- Iris:
  - Iris melanoma
  - Uveal melanoma

- Retina:
  - Retinoblastoma
  - Retinal haemangioma
  - Retinal astrocytoma

Incidence

- Metastatic lesions to the eye and the surrounding orbit are the most common orbital tumours in adults:
  - The choroid is a frequent site for metastasis of extra-ocular tumours due to its highly vascular nature
  - Primary neoplasias arise most often from breast, lung, gastrointestinal (GI) tract, kidney, and prostate
  - Metastases may be multiple and present in both eyes
- Melanoma of the uveal tract, particularly the choroid and ciliary body, is the most common primary intra-ocular malignancy of adults:
  - Usually unilateral and singular in nature
  - The incidence is approximately six to eight cases per million people per year
  - Uveal tract melanoma primarily affects adults 60 to 70 years of age; however, there is also a lesser peak incidence in the third decade of life
  - Caucasions have a tenfold greater risk. More frequent in people with fair skin complexion. There may be a genetic predisposition
  - The tumour is rare in the paediatric population
- Retinoblastoma is the most common paediatric primary eye neoplasm

Melanoma presentation

- Melanoma is a potentially lethal disease that has polymorphic presentation
- Primary ocular melanoma is particularly insidious
- Frequently painless and otherwise asymptomatic in early stages
- Often first suspected upon routine ophthalmologic examination
- Presenting symptoms depend on the location and size of the tumour:
  - Large neoplasias near the macula may produce early visual changes
  - Often uveal melanomas do not produce early symptoms. For example, ciliary body melanomas can grow behind the iris and may fail to be discovered until very late stage

Prognosis

Prognosis is dependent upon:
- Size:
  - Tumour size at the time of diagnosis is a strong predictor of ultimate tumour-related mortality
  - Smaller masses are less likely to have metastasized than larger tumours and thus have a more favourable prognosis
  - Five-year mortality for large tumours is 50%, up to 30% for medium-sized tumours, and 6–12% for small choroidal primary melanomas
- Histopathology:
  - Spindle-shaped melanoma cells have a better prognosis than epithelioid-shaped cells

- Most uveal tract melanomas have a mixture of both cell types and thus an intermediate prognosis

Mortality

- Left untreated or undiagnosed, it can metastasize from the eye and ultimately be fatal
- Most frequent sites for metastasis include liver, lung, and bone
- Median survival rate with metastatic disease is less than one year

Clinical interventions for melanoma

Surgical biopsy of an ocular lesion may lead to permanent impairment of vision and/or metastasis of tumour, so often diagnosis is dependent upon indirect tests and imaging studies such as ophthalmoscopy, fluorescein angiography, fundus photography, ultrasound, computed tomography (CT) scan, and magnetic resonance imaging (MRI). Once a finding of ocular melanoma is reached, a thorough investigation for metastatic disease is warranted to determine the optimal treatment plan.

There are several modalities of intervention:

- Enucleation:
  - The traditional means of therapy
  - Best option for large tumours or those with extracapsular extension
  - Definitive, provided there are no extra-ocular metastases
- Iridectomy or choroidectomy:
  - Rare options
- Radiation therapy:
  - External proton beam therapy (teletherapy)
  - Surgical implantation of radioactive seeds anchored to the globe (brachytherapy)
- Chemotherapy
- Photocoagulation
- Cryotherapy

There is controversy as to optimal approach for primary choroidal and ciliary body tumours.

- Proponents of enucleation believe that excision of the globe provides definitive and curative treatment. They argue that alternative therapies may preserve vision at the risk of patients' lives
- Advocates of newer globe-salvaging therapies point out that such treatment may preserve both the globe and vision, and result in enhanced quality of life without increased morbidity. Some ophthalmologists argue that surgical manipulation of the globe during enucleation may result in metastases and increased morbidity

The majority of larger- and medium-sized primary ocular melanomas are treated by enucleation. Small choroidal tumours are observed until there is evidence of change in the nature of the mass. Some ophthalmologists, however, believe that early intervention may ultimately result in overall improved survival of patients with small masses.

Whichever treatment modality is ultimately proven more beneficial, in the operating theatre the anaesthetist must be prepared to encounter patients with the same disease undergoing vastly different surgical procedures.

The perioperative concerns, anaesthetic implications, and management of melanoma patients differ markedly for patients undergoing enucleation versus surgically placed radiation therapy.

Enucleation

Patients with primary intra-ocular melanoma who elect to have enucleation come to the operating theatre anticipating a single definitive operation. In some countries, the majority of these cases are scheduled as ambulatory procedures with the patient discharged from the facility within a few hours following surgery, whilst in others overnight stay is more common.

Patients usually present to theatre with heightened levels of anxiety as:

- The eye scheduled to be removed often retains all or most visual function
- The diagnosis of cancer was established by indirect means, leading to a modicum of uncertainty
- Fear of potential life-threatening secondary spread of tumour
- Prior to surgery, anxiolytic medications may be quite beneficial
- Benzodiazepines are the agents of choice and may be administered orally or intravenously

Anaesthetic options

Enucleation of the globe can be accomplished under either GA or RA. The age range of the majority of patients with primary ocular melanoma is between 60 and 70 years old, so anaesthetic considerations for dealing with geriatric patients must be considered (see 📖 General anaesthesia aspects, pp. 192–195). These include age-related alterations of cardiac, pulmonary, renal, hepatic, and CNS system functions. Concomitant issues such as coronary artery disease, hypertension, diabetes, and osteoarthritis may influence the selection of anaesthetics and choice of anaesthetic technique.

General anaesthesia

- Minimum alveolar concentration of anaesthetic agents declines with age, producing diminished dose requirements for both induction and maintenance of anaesthesia
- The airway can be secured with a supraglottic device such as a LMA. An endotracheal tube may be preferable in the face of history of active gastrooesophageal reflux
- Anaesthesia can be maintained with inhalational or total intravenous techniques
- Neuromuscular paralysis is not necessary
- Oculo-cardiac reflex (see 📖 Oculo-cardiac reflex pp. 44–45):
  - Very commonly encountered
  - Manifests as a sudden bradycardia
  - May lead to full asystolic cardiac arrest
  - Exacerbated by hypoxaemia, hypercarbia, and light planes of anaesthesia
  - May occur with pressure on the empty socket after the globe has been removed
  - Management relies upon having the surgeon cease the precipitating stimulus, usually traction on an extra-ocular muscle or pressure placed within the orbit
  - Anticholinergics reverse and block further bradycardia. Atropine should be carefully considered prior to use in geriatric patients with coronary heart disease as the ensuing tachycardia may precipitate ischemia
  - Local anaesthetic injection may prevent further recurrence, although, paradoxically the block may itself induce an OCR
  - The reflex tends to attenuate and fatigue (tachyphylaxis)

- Postoperative nausea and vomiting:
  - High incidence
  - Postulated oculo-gastric reflex
  - Routine administration of prophylactic antiemetics may be prudent
- Postoperative pain management:
  - Narcotics may contribute to postoperative nausea and vomiting
  - NSAIDs are appropriate
  - Ophthalmic regional block prior to emergence from GA or immediately after induction (pre-emptive analgesia)

Regional anaesthesia

When combined with intravenous sedation, RA is a suitable alternative to GA.

- Requires a dense motor and sensory block of prolonged duration
- Epinephrine admixed into the LA lengthens and intensifies effect. It produces vasoconstriction that may decrease intraoperative bleeding. However, systemic absorption via the nasal mucosa may induce hypertension, tachydysrhythmia, or myocardial ischemia
- There is a high incidence of PONV and routine administration of prophylactic antiemetics is helpful
- Postoperative pain management is achieved by administration of long-acting LAs (bupivacaine, ropivacaine) for the initial block and supplemented by NSAID agents

Amnesia is a principal benefit provided by GA. Intraoperative awareness and recall are not the key issues for patients undergoing cataract extraction and lens implantation but they are foremost factors in enucleation surgery conducted under RA. One seeks to prevent any intraoperative recall, particularly when the thick, stout optic nerve is transected in the last step prior to removing the globe from the orbit by generous use of sedatives. Routine deep sedation is relatively contraindicated for most ophthalmologic procedures since potential abrupt head movements associated with changing levels of anaesthetic depth or responses by the patient to airway obstruction may place the eye and vision at risk. The need for amnesia and ablation of awareness outweighs these factors for patients undergoing globe enucleation, since jeopardizing the eye is not an issue.

Postoperative care

An analysis of postoperative complications of large choroidal melanoma enucleation surgery without distinction as to type of anaesthesia. In order of frequency, postoperative problems were pain, nausea/vomiting, and haemorrhage. Less commonly, cardiovascular and pulmonary issues, urinary retention, and fever were reported.

Radioactive seed implantation

Surgical implantation of radioactive seeds (brachytherapy) consists of surgical anchoring of a plaque embedded with radioactive seeds onto the sclera in proximity to the melanoma. The plaque is shielded with gold or similar material on one side such that the radiation is focused directly at the lesion, with minimal radioactive exposure to surrounding unaffected tissue (see Figure 18.1).

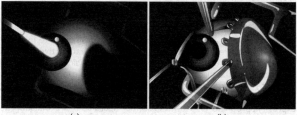

(a)	(b)

Fig. 18.1 (a): intra-ocular tumour transilluminated by light through pupil.
(b): *in-situ* shielded plaque. Illustrations by Jennifer Thomson, Bascom Palmer Eye Institute, University of Miami Miller School of Medicine.

There are a number of distinctions between globe enucleation and the surgical placement of a radioactive plaque for treatment of intraocular melanoma. The former is usually accomplished as a single procedure, whilst the latter requires two operations (placement and subsequent removal of the seeds). The duration of surgery for both the application of the radioactive plaque and its later removal is brief.

Plaque placement

Patients usually present to theatre with less anxiety than enucleation patients. Anxiolytic medications may nonetheless be of assistance.

Anaesthetic options

In contrast to enucleation, the great majority of patients undergoing episcleral plaque radiotherapy receive regional anaesthesia.
- Needle or cannula-based injection of LA is appropriate. Topical anaesthesia is inadequate due to the extensive manipulation of the globe associated with surgical placement of the plaque
- Liberal use of intravenous sedation is permissible as surgery is extra-ocular

Severe claustrophobia or surgeon's preference is the most common indications for GA. It is important to maintain normocarbia with adequate ventilation for patients under GA. Hypoventilation and resulting hypercarbia may increase choroidal blood flow, making surgery more formidable.

Postoperative care

For patients who have had a GA, an ophthalmic regional block given intra-operatively provides postoperative pain management. Use of long-acting LAs (bupivacaine, ropivacaine) is helpful. Regional block is supplemented with NSAIDs.

The incidence of PONV is very high due to external pressure on the globe by the plaque. It is important to consider routine administration of prophylactic antiemetics or rescue antiemetics should be readily available.

Plaque removal

The removal of the plaque usually takes less than 15–20min.

Many brachytherapy patients remain as inpatients in order to minimize radiation exposure to others and to assure that no radioactive materials are lost. The theoretical possibility of a radioactive iodine seed becoming dislodged from the plaque and displaced outside the eye exists. Patients frequently express frustration at the restriction of free movement during the three days of inpatient status. Anaesthesia and other personnel must express appropriate empathy. Anxiolytic medications are helpful. The plaque and inflammation may be painful. Analgesics may be indicated.

Anaesthesia options

Patients undergoing surgical removal of a plaque have the equivalent of a space-occupying intra-orbital mass consisting of the radioactive plaque itself, surgical materials, and local tissue inflammation. Tissue engorgement is a response to the recent surgical manipulation, presence of the foreign body, and effect of radiation. This expansion of intra-orbital mass markedly reduces the extra-global free volume within the orbit, thus diminishing the potential space for LAs.

- Sub-Tenon's block is less effective because conjunctiva and Tenon's capsule have been disrupted. There may be difficulty in negotiating the blunt cannula posteriorly. There is more pronounced forward reflux of LAs
- Extraconal (peribulbar) block requires higher volumes of LA agent, but there may be insufficient space to inject even the minimal required amount
- Traditional approach intraconal (retrobulbar) block, the needle directed posteriorly with low volume of LA agent may be most suitable
- Oculocardiac reflex incidence is quite frequent and pronounced
- Atropine should be readily available
- Quality of analgesia may be less adequate, requiring supplementation with additional block and/or deeper levels of sedation
- GA may be indicated in the face of inadequate block analgesia

Postoperative care

Postoperative pain management is usually not a problem. Ophthalmic block performed as a primary method of anaesthesia provides sufficient pain relief. However, a NSAID should be supplemented.

The incident of PONV is low due to relief of pressure on the globe. However, rescue antiemetics should be prescribed.

Clinical interventions for retinoblastoma

Children with retinoblastoma require frequent examinations under anaesthesia (EUA) to closely monitor the disease and recognize its progression and complications in a timely fashion.

- Retinoblastoma accounts for:
  - Almost 1% of all paediatric cancer deaths
  - Nearly 3% of all childhood cancers
  - 5% of cases of childhood blindness
  - Third most common intra-ocular cancer overall after melanoma and metastasis
  - 90% present before 3 years of age
  - 60% unilateral, 40% bilateral
- Presenting symptoms usually include leukocoria and strabismus:
  - Typically leukocoria is noted upon physical examination by the paediatrician
  - Parents note a white reflection in the baby's eye(s) in photographs
- Genetic considerations:
  - Lack or malfunction of the *Rb* gene on the long arm of chromosome 13
  - Gene functions to prevent formation of neoplasias in healthy individuals
  - The first tumour-suppressing function gene discovered
  - Since every cell is missing the gene, tumours can form in one or both eyes
  - There is a non-heritable form of retinoblastoma—a single cell's *Rb* gene is affected during development, thus tumour only emerges unilaterally
- Treatment options include:
  - Enucleation
  - Laser therapy
  - Radiation
  - Chemotherapy
  - Combined modalities (laser, radiation, chemotherapy)

Enucleation is reserved for children with extensive disease or those who have not responded to globe-salvaging therapies. The majority of patients, however, come to theatre for minimally invasive procedures. Quite often there is no actual surgery on the day of surgery. Interventions in the operating room include:

- Detailed fundoscopic examination
- Photography
- Ultrasound
- Laser photocoagulation
- Cryotherapy
- Thermotherapy

Preoperative considerations

Children may return to the operating theatre quite regularly over the course of their early childhood due to the need to follow progression/regression of the disease and provide therapy on a continuing basis.

- Psychosocial considerations for both patient and parents should not be ignored
- Small children may begin to fear trips to the hospital:
  - 'White-coat' or 'blue-scrubs' syndrome
- Age-appropriate preoperative tours of the operating theatre and/or explanatory videos for home-viewing may allay day-of-surgery anxieties
- Establish a family- and child-centric waiting area:
  - Casual, relaxed atmosphere
  - Ample interesting toys
  - Childrens' video programmes
- Consider anxiolytic premedications:
  - Midazolam 0.2–0.4mg/kg up to 20mg maximum
- Preoperative laboratory investigations:
  - Generally unnecessary
  - Consider a complete blood count for children who have had recent chemotherapy

Anaesthetic considerations

- A smooth and atraumatic induction of general anaesthesia reduces incidence of postoperative dysphoria and long-term emotional squeal
- Anaesthesia can be inhalational or ketamine-based
- Parental presence at induction of inhalational anaesthesia is controversial:
  - Can allay childrens' anxiety
  - Little impact for infants
  - Some parents may be distressed by the foreign environment
- Inhalation induction with sevoflurane:
  - Circumvents childrens' natural aversion to needles
  - Favourable cardiovascular profile
  - Lack of respiratory irritation compared to other inhaled anaesthetic agents
  - Alternatively, consider intravenous or intramuscular ketamine for induction if intra-ocular pressure assessment is included in the planned EUA
- Rendell–Baker mask:
  - Mask edge is tapered away from the eyes
  - Improves eye accessibility for the ophthalmologist, photographer, and ultrasonographer
  - May be difficult to establish a good mask seal
- Intravenous cannulation:
  - May forgo if brief procedure is anticipated and patient at low risk of aspiration, laryngospasm etc. The insertion of an intravenous cannula at some stage during the procedure is considered essential in many countries
  - Maintain airway with a facemask or LMA

- Assure adequate depth of anaesthesia prior to any manipulation of the eye to preclude episodes of laryngospasm or oculocardiac reflex
- Atropine, epinephrine, and suxamethonium doses should be calculated, prepared, and made immediately available for intramuscular administration in the absence of an intravenous line should bradycardia or laryngospasm occur
- Good communication between the ophthalmologists, technicians, and anaesthetists is a key component in ensuring suitable anaesthesia care
- If actual surgery or multiple procedures are planned, place an IV cannula and secure the airway with a laryngeal mask or endotracheal tube
- Bell's phenomenon:
  - Eyes gaze upward as lids begin to close
  - A natural protective reflex
  - Indicator of depth of anaesthesia
  - With light plane of anaesthesia, the globe turns cephalad in response to pressure on the eye by the lid speculum
  - With deep plane of anaesthesia, the reflex is extinguished, and the eye remains in neutral gaze

Postoperative care
- Emergence delirium:
  - Post-sevoflurane agitation
  - May be more common in children with heightened levels of preoperative anxiety
  - Not due to pain
  - More frequent in children under 6 years old
  - May be ameliorated by midazolam, propofol, narcotics, or NSAIDs
- Postoperative pain management: pain is minimal but intravenous, intramuscular or rectal paracetomol may help
- PONV may occur

Conclusion

Ocular tumours are often painless and otherwise asymptomatic in their earlier stages. Without treatment, there is potential for vision loss, or with metastasis, they can be fatal. The two entities most commonly encountered in the operating theatre are uveal tract melanoma and retinoblastoma. Traditional forms of treatment such as enucleation are being supplanted by newer globe-salvaging techniques. Anaesthetists must be aware of the anaesthetic implications of ocular tumours.

Key reading

Parrish RK (ed.)*The University of Miami Bascom Palmer Eye Institute atlas of ophthalmology*, 2nd edn. Oxford: Butterworth-Heinemann, 2000.

Chapter 19

Anaesthesia for ocular trauma

Mr Brian C. Baumann and Dr Ashish Sinha

Introduction

Controversies exist regarding the optimal anaesthetic management of patients requiring surgery for ocular trauma. Ocular injuries are commonly encountered in clinical practice and an estimated 750,000 patients are hospitalized with eye injuries annually throughout the world. Many, particularly those with open globe injuries, require surgery, often under emergency conditions that make the patient's anaesthetic management challenging.

This chapter reviews epidemiological data illustrating the prevalence and incidence of serious eye injuries and then presents a case study detailing the anaesthetic management of a severely traumatized patient to illustrate a discussion of current options and recommendations for the management of such cases.

Epidemiology of traumatic eye injuries

Epidemiology of traumatic eye injuries

Traumatic eye injuries are a common problem that can occur in the workplace, at home, during leisure activities such as sports, or as a result of road accidents or assault. Estimates of the incidence, prevalence, and seriousness of such injuries are imprecise because of the methodological limitations of the available epidemiological studies that usually rely on population surveys or reviews of hospital records.

Eye trauma is generally believed to be more common and more serious in developing countries, but the developed world is not spared.

- A survey of more than 5,000 urban residents over the age of 40 in one American city revealed that 22.5% of black males, 20.3% of white males, 12.2% of black females, and 7.7% of white females recalled having experienced ocular trauma for a cumulative lifetime prevalence rate of 14,300 injuries for every 100,000 people
- A similarly sized survey of urban and rural residents of Australia over the age of 40 revealed that 34.2% of males and 9.9% of females reported having had an ocular injury that required medical attention
- These self-reported prevalence rates are even higher than those reported in a survey of almost 40,000 Nepalese that revealed that 1,780 of every 100,000 people either had clinical evidence of traumatic eye injury or reported a history of ocular injury before age 60
- The World Health Organization (WHO) estimated that globally there were 55 million eye injuries annually that restricted the patient's activity for at least one day
- In the US alone, there were at least 2.5 million such traumatic eye injuries annually
- The incidence of ocular trauma can also vary dramatically over time as the introduction of new industries into a region can increase the risk of occupational injury while advances in prevention, such as seatbelts and protective eyewear, can reduce the incidence of serious eye injury
- In addition to the morbidity associated with these ocular injuries, there are also large financial costs
- In the US, the total annual cost to society associated with ophthalmic trauma is estimated to be greater than US$4 billion (€ 2.9 billion)

Fortunately, most eye injuries are minor or self-limiting and can be treated successfully in outpatient facilities, but the WHO estimates that worldwide some 750,000 of these injuries resulted in hospitalization.

- In the industrialized world, the estimated incidence of eye injuries requiring hospitalization was 13 per 100,000 population per year, but methodological inconsistencies in the reported epidemiological studies contribute to rates of hospitalization that vary widely from country to country and even within countries
- Studies have reported annual incidence rates for hospitalization due to traumatic ocular injury per 100,000 populations of 8.1 for Scotland, 15.2 for Sweden, 4.9 for Italy, and 12.6 for Singapore
- One Australian study estimated an annual incidence of 15.2 admissions per 100,000 while another Australian study reported an annual rate of 57 hospitalizations per 100,000

- Estimates of admission for ocular trauma in the US ranged from 4.1 to 13.2 per 100,000 populations
- One Australian study reported that 8% of ocular trauma required hospitalization in contrast to two British studies in which only 0.9% and 1.8%, respectively, of traumatic eye injuries required admission

Traumatic injuries resulting in hospitalization can be broadly categorized as either 'open globe' injuries in which the integrity of the ocular wall is breached versus 'closed globe' injuries in which the ocular wall remains intact.

- Open globe injuries such as ruptures, lacerations or penetrating wounds are of particular importance to anaesthetists because these injuries usually require surgery, often emergency procedures under conditions that complicate the anaesthetic management of the patient
- Ten years ago, the WHO estimated that there were 200,000 annual admissions worldwide for such open globe injuries
- In the US, as in the rest of the world, the problem is particularly common among males whose risk ranges from 6 to 9 times higher than the risk for females. In the US Eye Injury Register database, 81% of serious trauma cases were males
- Risk peaks for males between ages 15–24 with some evidence of a secondary increase in incidence for older males, possibly because of an increased risk of blunt trauma globe rupture as a result of a prior history of having had a large-incision cataract extraction, corneal transplant, glaucoma filtering procedures, or laser *in-situ* keratomileusis (LASIK). In contrast, the risk of trauma peaks for females between ages 5–14

Epidemiological studies suggest that the annual incidence of open globe traumatic injuries is approximately 3.5 cases per 100,000 populations.

- An annual incidence of 3.6 per 100,000 was reported from Australia while a rate of 3.0 per 100,000 per year was reported in a two-decade retrospective hospital-based study in Germany
- Researchers in Stockholm reported an annual incidence of 6.0 per 100,000 males and a corresponding incidence of 1.2 for females. Review of hospital records for well-defined populations in the US found the incidence of perforating eye traumas per 100,000 populations to be 2 in Wisconsin and 3.8 in Maryland

Ocular traumas, particularly open globe injuries, are a source of serious morbidity.

- A WHO survey estimated that 1.6 million people worldwide have been blinded in both eyes by trauma. An additional 2.3 million individuals have bilateral low vision while 19 million people have monocular blindness or low vision caused by traumatic injuries
- In the US, estimates are that the prevalence of bilateral blindness from trauma is 9 per 100,000 populations, affecting at least 19,400 individuals. The same study estimated that nearly 1 million Americans had permanent visual impairment from trauma with more than 75% of these having monocular blindness. Trauma was second only to cataracts as a cause of visual impairment in the US population with 50,000 new cases of traumatic visual impairment reported each year. In a population survey from an American city, 21.2 of every 1000 black

males over age 40 had monocular blindness from prior trauma, a prevalence even higher than that observed in Nepal where 8.6 of every 1000 residents had traumatic monocular blindness

• Open globe injuries are often associated with concurrent injuries to the head, orbit, and adnexa, especially in cases of blunt force trauma. In a study of 300 patients with open globe injuries, orbital, and adnexal injuries were observed in 25.7% of patients, with peri-ocular lacerations, orbital fracture, and retrobulbar haemorrhage the most common

Surgical management and outcomes

These open globe injuries can often be managed successfully with surgery, which is more commonly performed in the community setting rather than in trauma centres.

- The definitive therapy for such injuries is rapid primary closure, usually within 24h of the injury, with antibiotic treatment to prevent endophthalmitis
- Surgery may preserve vision in up to 75% of patients, the outcome dependent primarily upon the degree of injury to the posterior segment of the globe
- The introduction of pars plana vitrectomy and improved antibiotic management of potential infection has increased the probability of functional success with surgical intervention
- Even for patients lacking any light perception in the traumatized eye, the US Eye Injury Register reported that 16% improved and 2% even achieved 20/40 or better visual acuity. The same survey found that among patients who still had light perception after their injury, 69% improved with surgery with 19% achieving normal visual acuity
- The prognosis for ruptured globe or for those with severe penetrating injuries is more disappointing with more than half of these eyes remaining blind and 12–21% requiring enucleation
- There is some hope for salvaging vision even after relatively severe injuries as a recent review reported that 40% of 109 eyes with penetrating injuries or ruptured globes had a good outcome with surgical intervention, achieving a final visual acuity score of 6/12 or better on the Snellen scale

Case study of the anaesthetic management of severe ophthalmic trauma

The following case study illustrates the approach to some of the many challenges in the anaesthetic management of patients with severe ocular injuries.

• An 18-year-old female presented with a severe open globe injury due to lacerations caused by shards from a helmet that shattered in a motorcycle accident, which occured three hours ago

• After examination in the emergency room, she was scheduled for an emergency exploration of her wound

• GA was induced using lidocaine (1mg/kg), fentanyl (2mcg/kg), propofol (2mg/kg) and suxamethonium (2mg/kg) to achieve a rapid sequence induction. Prior to the administration of suxamethonium, a defasciculating dose of vecuronium (0.01mg/kg) was given. A size 7 endotracheal tube was placed uneventfully. After spontaneous recovery from suxamethonium, a paralyzing dose of vecuronium was administered (0.1mg/kg). Anaesthetic state was maintained with desflurane (6%) in a mixture of oxygen and air

• Following completion of the 4h procedure, which included enucleation and placement of an ocular prosthesis, paralysis was reversed in the presence of one twitch out of four with neostigmine (0.07mg/kg) and glycopyrrolate. An IV dose of lidocaine was administered prior to extubation to attenuate the sympathetic response to extubation

• After the patient regained spontaneous ventilation, she was kept in the lateral head-down position to decrease risk of aspiration, and the endotracheal tube was removed uneventfully

Five months after her emergency surgery, she presented for additional sinus surgery. Her anaesthetic management was handled routinely, and the case was completed uneventfully.

Like this young patient, many patients with open globe traumatic injuries require surgery. Successful surgical management requires the use of anaesthetic techniques that achieve akinesia, analgesia, attenuation of the oculocardiac reflex, control of IOP, minimal bleeding, and smooth emergence. Achieving these goals while maintaining patient safety as the highest priority poses some challenges.

• The risk of aspiration must be minimized, particularly since many patients requiring emergency surgery may have full stomachs

• Drugs must be selected prudently to minimize increases in IOP that could exacerbate the injury by causing extrusion of orbital contents

• The particular problems associated with anaesthesia for children and the very elderly, two groups with a relatively high incidence of ocular trauma, create additional challenges

• Successful management requires that all steps in the anaesthetic process be tailored specifically to the individual patient, including preoperative preparation, drug selection, airway management, maintenance of anaesthesia, extubation, and recovery.

Preoperative evaluation

Preoperatively, the patient must receive a comprehensive evaluation to determine the extent of all injuries so that the benefits of early closure of the ocular injury can be weighed against the risk of operating on a patient who may have significant traumatic injuries to other organs. The possibility that the patient may have abused alcohol or drugs should be assessed as these factors could influence the patient's response to a given dose of anaesthetic agents.

- Preoperatively, an attempt should also be made to assess the patient's NPO status to estimate the risk of aspiration as patients presenting for emergency surgery often have a full stomach. Alternatively, patients for urgent but not emergent eye surgery may have minimal risk for aspiration. Evacuation of gastric contents with a nasogastric tube is problematic since such a procedure may lead to coughing, gagging, or other responses that dramatically increase IOP.
- The patient's pulmonary status should be ascertained preoperatively: patients with decreased functional residual capacity become hypoxic more quickly, making a rapid induction technique preferable.
- The size of an ocular perforation should be assessed preoperatively as small punctures are less likely to have loss of vitreous material with increases in intra-ocular pressure compared to larger punctures.

Selecting the method of anaesthesia

Although needle-based ophthalmic RA and even topical anaesthesia with lidocaine combined with IV sedation has been used successfully in selected cases of open globe injuries and may be unavoidable for medically unstable patients, GA is often preferred for serious injuries in patients without contraindications.

Topical anaesthesia is not suitable for cases requiring ocular akinesia or significant intra-ocular manipulation.

Regional anaesthesia

RA can be administered with an intraconal (retrobulbar) block or extra-conal (peribulbar) needle injection.

- The standard anaesthetic solution consists of an equal mixture of 2% to 4% lidocaine and 0.75% bupivacaine with up to 15 units of hyaluronidase.
- Small amounts (<0.5cc) of anaesthetic should be injected slowly while visualizing the globe to monitor for concerning changes, particularly in the area of the wound.
- The block may later be supplemented with a sub-Tenon's block.
- In select cases, a lid block administered before the needle block may be appropriate.
- In a small Italian study, topical oxybuprocaine hydrochloride 0.4% combined with IV propofol, midazolam, and fentanyl for anaesthesia proved effective for less severe open globe injuries.

General anaesthesia for ocular trauma

Agents for reducing gastric acidity and the probability of vomiting

- Patients selected for GA may benefit from manoeuvres to reduce gastric acidity and/or the probability of vomiting
- Preoperative administration of metoclopramide (0.15mg/kg) given intravenously at the time of admission and continuing every 2–4h until surgery can reduce the risk of aspiration and increased IOP associated with emesis by accelerating gastric emptying
- Alternatively, a serotonin antagonist like ondansetron given intravenously provides comparable efficacy for prevention of emesis although without the advantage of accelerating gastric emptying
- Although H_2-histamine-receptor antagonists like ranitidine inhibit gastric acid secretion, their usefulness in emergency surgery is limited because they do not lower the pH of gastric secretions already present in the stomach
- Non-particulate antacids like sodium citrate have a more immediate pH-lowering effect, short 30–60min duration of action, and are most useful if administered just prior to induction to reduce gastric acidity in an effort to limit damage should aspiration occur
- More prolonged use of antacids for patients requiring emergency surgery is not recommended since these substances increase intra-gastric volume

neuromuscular blocker (e.g. vecuronium) and an appropriate dose of an anaesthetic, suxamethonium will cause only a small increase in IOP. This small increase is believed to be insignificant when compared to the increase in IOP that would result from the Valsalva response to intubation.

- As an alternative to suxamethonium, there are non-depolarizing paralytic agents such as the aminosteroids, specifically the fast-acting rocuronium, that avoid the risk of intra-ocular hypertension entirely in situations when emergent endotracheal intubation is necessary.
  A metanalysis of studies comparing suxamethonium with rocuronium for emergent intubation found that the clinical effectiveness of the two drugs was comparable, but suxamethonium more frequently created excellent intubating conditions and was able to achieve suitable intubating conditions slightly faster than rocuronium.
- Another non-depolarizing agent, vecuronium, has a slightly longer time to onset and a longer duration of action than rocuronium and is really not suitable for RSI.

Cricoid pressure

- Regardless of the choice of neuromuscular agent, it may be prudent to further reduce the risk of aspiration by having an assistant apply adequate external pressure over the cricoid ring until verification of tube placement and inflation of the endotracheal tube cuff is completed
- Controversy exists in the literature concerning the benefits of this practice
- There is limited evidence that external pressure on the cricoid reduces the incidence of aspiration, and some studies suggest it may contribute to airway obstruction and difficulty intubating
- However, until more definitive evidence is published, cricoid pressure is still considered mandatory during RSI

Supraglottic airway

GA for urgent/non-emergent surgery on patients not at substantive risk for aspiration may be accomplished with an LMA. Supraglottic airways offer the advantage of minimal impact on IOP upon placement and at emergence.

Maintenance of anaesthesia

Once induction has been achieved, anaesthesia can usually be maintained without difficulty by using an inhaled anaesthetic like desflurane or sevoflurane in a mixture of air and oxygen. Although neither of these agents exerts a direct effect on the IOP, both are associated with a 16–18% risk of postoperative vomiting that may cause a transient, potentially harmful elevation of IOP.

Alternatively, maintenance of anaesthesia can also be achieved with TIVA using propofol and remifentanil.

Extubation and emergence also present an increased risk of pulmonary aspiration and so must be accomplished when the patient is fully awake and has intact airway reflexes.

At this point, some recommend keeping the patient in the lateral head-down position until the tube is removed. In this patient population, this method of extubation has been applied frequently with no reports of extrusion of orbital contents.

If deep extubation is required, the risk of pulmonary aspiration can be reduced but not eliminated by intraoperative administration of antiemetics or nasogastric tube suctioning.

Chapter 20

Retained visual sensations during ophthalmic surgery under regional anaesthesia

Dr K.G. AuEong

Dr Tiakumzuk Sangtam

Introduction

Retained visual sensations are visual perceptions or experiences encountered by patients in their operated eye during surgical procedures. For the purpose of this chapter, the terms visual experience and visual perceptions will be used synonymously with retained visual sensations.

Effect of regional anaesthesia on optic nerve function

RA techniques such as intraconal (retrobulbar), extraconal (peribulbar) and sub-Tenon's blocks involve administration of a considerable volume of LA agents in a restricted compartment of the orbit. The effect of these local techniques on the optic nerve is variable, ranging from no light perception to diminished visual acuity, relative afferent pupillary defect and changes in visual evoked potentials. Several proposed mechanisms include:

- Transient conduction blockade of the optic nerve
- Relative ischaemia produced by compression from the volume of anaesthetic solution
- Saturation of the photoreceptor elements and the retinal pigment epithelium
- Blur induced by post-injection digital pressure
- Induced hyperopia through posterior globe indentation by the anaesthetic volume

Usual expressions of retained visual sensations during ophthalmic surgeries

A number of case reports and clinical studies have documented this phenomenon during cataract, glaucoma, vitreous, and LASIK surgeries. These include perception of:

- Light
- One or more colours
- Movements
- Flashes of light
- Instruments
- Surgeon's fingers or hands
- Change in light brightness

The visual images seen by each patient are unique (see Table 20.1) because they are a combination of images of objects close to but outside the eye (e.g., fingers, hands, instruments) and entoptic phenomena produced by objects and structures on the corneal surface and in the eye.

Table 20.1 Intraoperative visual sensations during cataract surgery under local anaesthesia

Type of cataract surgery	Extra-capsular cataract extraction	Phacoemulsification		
Type of anaesthesia	Retrobulbar	Retrobulbar	Peribulbar	Sub-Tenon's	Topical
Proportion of patients who perceived:					
No light (%)	4–20	9.3–15.7	–	12.5–19	0–26.5
Light (%)	80–96	84.3–90.7	80.9	81–87.8	89.7–100
Movements (%)	39–68	34.7–48.6	–	35.5–40	18.6–61.5
Flashes (%)	36–66	43.3–50	–	4	6.9–60.2
Colour(s) (%)	56–80	55.7–61.3	49	56–56.8	69.6–96.2
Instruments (%)	16–73.1	17.1–18	15.9	7–10.8	0–37.1
Surgeon's hands/fingers (%)	10	15.7	–	10–12.5	0–29.6
Surgeon/medical staff (%)	–	13.3	–	4.8	7.1–9.1
Change in light brightness (%)	44–64	44.3–51.3	–	11.5–39	46.2–92.5

Dynamic factors such as moving fluids and bubbles on the corneal surface and in the eye as well as moving instruments in the eye also add to the changing kaleidoscope of colours and shapes reported by many patients.

During cataract surgery under topical anaesthesia, the ever-changing shape and opacity of the lens as it is being emulsified, aspirated or extracted as well as changes in the refractive state of the eye from phakic, to initially aphakic, and finally pseudophakic state also influence the focusing of light rays on the retina and hence the visual sensations.

Likewise, deformation of the cornea, the main refractive element of the eye, such as during expression of the lens nucleus in extracapsular cataract extraction (ECCE), lifting of the LASIK corneal flap, and excimer laser treatment on the cornea can also create visual images.

Glaucoma patients undergoing trabeculectomy, phacotrabeculectomy or glaucoma tube implantation using RA see images similar to those experienced by patients during cataract extraction (see Table 20.2).

Table 20.2 Intraoperative visual sensations during glaucoma surgery (trabeculectomy, phacotrabeculectomy, tube implants) under peribulbar anaesthesia

Visual sensation	Proportion of patients perceiving visual sensation (%)
No light throughout surgery	13.3–26.7
Light	73.3–86.7
Movements	42.7–65
Flashes	53.3
One or more colours	48.3–61.3
Instruments	8.3–41.3
Surgeon's hand/fingers	44
Surgeon/medical staff	1.7
Change in light brightness	38.3–60

Differences in retained visual sensations during phacoemulsification under topical versus regional anaesthesia

Patients undergoing phacoemulsification under topical anaesthesia are more aware of their visual environment than those operated under RA. In RCTs comparing topical with RA, more patients under topical anaesthesia perceived light, colours (including more colours at the early stages of phacoemulsification and more blue throughout surgery) and changes in light brightness when compared to those operated on under RA.

Differences in retained visual sensations between glaucoma and cataract surgeries

Although the findings of different clinical series are not directly comparable, a relatively higher proportion of glaucoma patients (41.3 to 44.0%) see complex, formed images such as surgical instruments and surgeon's hands or fingers compared with patients undergoing phacoemulsification here 7.0 to 26.1% can see instruments and 10.0 to 25.0% perceive the surgeon's hands or fingers. These differences may be explained in part by the location of the surgical instruments in the different procedures: predominantly extra-ocular during glaucoma surgery versus anterior chamber or anterior segment during cataract surgery. It is possible that surgical instruments in the anterior segment are not seen as clearly as those outside the eye. In addition, compared to cataract surgery in which the crystalline lens is disrupted or removed by manipulation and phacoemulsification rendering the eye aphakic initially and subsequently pseudophakic after implantation of an IOL, a purely glaucoma surgery usually does not disturb the optical elements of the eye and therefore the refractive status remains relatively unchanged, thus enabling the patient to better perceive objects outside the eye.

Furthermore, glaucoma patients perceive fluctuating light intensity in 60% of cases. This fluctuation may be explained by variation in the intensity of the operating microscope light by shadows cast from the surgeon's hands, fingers or surgical instruments, and by the relative movements of the eye during different parts of the surgery.

Retained visual sensations during vitreous surgery

In general, retained visual sensations during vitreous surgery under regional (either intra- or extraconal) anaesthesia are less common when compared to that during cataract surgery (see Table 20.3). This could be attributable to the greater volume of anaesthetic agent commonly used during vitreous surgery as well as the presence of more severe pre-existing retinal pathology.

Table 20.3 Intraoperative visual sensations during vitreous surgery under regional (retrobulbar, peribulbar or sub-Tenon's) anaesthesia

Visual sensation	Proportion of patients experiencing visual sensation (%)
No light perception throughout surgery	10–24.6
Transient no light perception	29.2
Light	46.2–90.1
Movements	55.4–63.8
Flashes	30–40
One or more colour	56.2–72.3
Instruments	47.5–53.5
Surgeon's hand/fingers	8.9–24.6
Surgeon/medical staff	3.1
Branching patterns of retinal blood vessels	21.5
Whirling black spots during triamcinolone-assisted vitrectomy	37.2

There is a significant correlation with the preoperative or postoperative visual acuity. Patients who report intraoperative sensation for not only light but also colours or moving objects, which are perceived mainly by the cone system, show significantly better postoperative visual acuity. In other words, the intraoperative visual sensations are correlated with the macular function of the patient.

Retained visual sensations during LASIK

Patients undergoing LASIK whether using microkeratome or femtosecond laser may see flashes, various colours, movements, the surgeon's hands or fingers and the surgeon during surgery (see Table 20.4). Interestingly, during both vacuum suction and corneal flap fashioning, a higher proportion of eyes using microkeratome lose light perception compared to eyes using femtosecond laser.

Table 20.4 Intraoperative visual sensations during LASIK under topical anaesthesia

Visual sensation	Proportion of patients perceiving visual sensation (%)
No light	39–90.2[*]
Light	100
Movements	86.6
Flashes	12.2
One or more colours	100
Instruments	92.7
Surgeon's hand/fingers	37.8
Surgeon/medical staff	2.4
Corneal flap being lifted	56.1
Red fixation light increasing in size	59.8
Red fixation light moving	37.8

[*]During application of suction and corneal flap fashioning.

Other expressions of retained visual sensations

Drawings and poetic expressions of intraoperative visual images during ophthalmic surgery

A number of patients including artists and even a poet have documented their visual experiences during different ophthalmic surgeries in the form of poetry, drawings and painting (see Poem 1).

Poem

Only rarely seen in dreams
Wondrous light from laser beams
To show such strong dramatic scenes
Only rarely seen dreams
This helps the eye to see

Bright and beautiful coils of light
Crystal clear to heal the sight
Soft and warm and glowing bright
Fascinating mystery

Subtle shades of pink and blue
Smoky white and yellow too
Will these show the same for you
As they did for me?

Our thanks to those who show the light
Their skills and loving care delight
And much improve our failing sight
A wondrous place to be

Work by a poet inspired by his visual experience during cataract surgery under local anaesthesia. (Reprinted with permission from: Zia R, Schlichtenbrede FC, Greaves B, Saeed MU (2005). "Only rarely seen in dreams"—visual experiences during cataract surgery. Br J Ophthalmol, **89**(2):247–8).

If 'a picture is worth a thousand words', the following pictures (see Figures 20.1, 20.2 and 20.3) are telling illustrations of the varied and elaborate visual sensations encountered during ophthalmic surgeries.

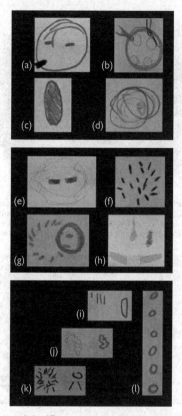

Fig. 20.1 Sketches made by different patients on their visual experience during cataract surgery under local anaesthesia. (Reprinted with permission from: Au Eong KG (2002). 6th Yahya Cohen Lecture: Visual experience during cataract surgery. Ann Acad Med Singapore, **31**(5):666–74).

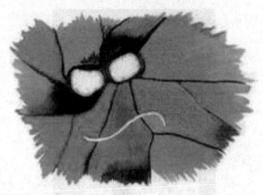

Fig. 20.2 "Colourful monkey"- an artist's impression of his visual experiences during cataract surgery under local anaesthesia. (Reprinted with permission from: Zia R, Schlichtenbrede FC, Greaves B, Saeed MU (2005). "Only rarely seen in dreams"—visual experiences during cataract surgery. *Br J Ophthalmol*, **89**(2):247–8).

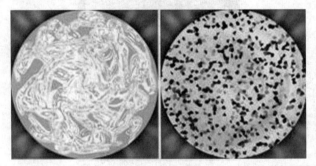

Fig. 20.3 Drawings by an artist inspired by his visual images during vitrectomy. (Left panel) The drawing depicts what he saw during vitrectomy when he reported seeing colorless swirling fluid. (Right panel) The drawing of the artist's perceptions of numerous black and grey spots like snowflakes most likely corresponding to intravitreal injection of white triamcinolone acetonide crystals. (Reprinted with permission from: Kawaguchi N, Inoue M, Sugimura E, et al (2006). Subjective visual sensation during vitrectomy under retrobulbar anesthesia. *Am J Ophthalmol*, **141**(2):407–9).

Pleasant versus unpleasant retained visual sensations

Retained visual sensations during ophthalmic surgeries can be unpleasant. Some patients even find them outright frightening (see Table 20.5). Interestingly, only 1.3% to 1.7% of glaucoma patients find their visual experience frightening compared with up to 16.2% of cataract patients. It is expected that many glaucoma patients undergoing surgery have glaucomatous optic nerve dysfunction and have undergone repeated glaucoma directed investigations involving complex instruments such as optic disc imaging, visual field testing, and retinal tomography. They may also have undergone previous laser procedures where there is exposure to a different light stimulus. Therefore, they may have less vivid visual sensations and are more familiar and comfortable with the various visual sensations and thus less likely to be afraid.

Table 20.5 Proportion of patients who find their intraoperative visual sensations during ophthalmic surgery frightening

Ophthalmic surgery	Type of anaesthesia	Proportion of patients who experienced fear (%)	Associations with a frightening visual experience
Cataract surgery	Retrobulbar	5–9.3	Colours, flashes of light, female gender
	Peribulbar	11.1	
	Sub-Tenon's	3–16.2	Colours, photophobia, volume of anaesthetic <4ml
	Topical	0–15.4	
Glaucoma surgery (trabeculectomy, phacotrabeculectomy, tube implants)	Peribulbar	1.3–1.7	
Vitreous surgery	Peribulbar/ retrobulbar	5.9–13.8	<65 years, longer surgery, colours
LASIK	Topical	19.5	First eye surgery

Clinical significance of retained visual sensations

The anxiety and fear that may result can cause patients to become unco-operative during the procedure or trigger a sympathetic stress response. This may result in hypertension, tachycardia, ischaemic strain on the heart, hyperventilation, and acute panic attacks. These stress responses are particularly undesirable in cataract patients who are often elderly and have systemic comorbidities such as diabetes, hypertension, and ischaemic heart disease. The frightening experience may also decrease patient satisfaction with the surgery.

Unless patients are counselled, the majority of them either expect to perceive nothing at all during cataract surgery or are unsure of what to expect (see Table 20.6).

Table 20.6 Proportion of patients who expect and experience visual sensations during phacoemulsification under topical anaesthesia

Visual sensation	Proportion of patients who expect visual sensation during surgery (%)	Proportion of patients who experience visual sensation during surgery (%)
Light	36.7	100
Colour(s)	18.4	81.6
Movements	20.4	55.1
Flashes	20.4	60.2
Instruments	8.2	21.4
Surgeon's fingers/hands	17.3	29.6
Surgeon/medical staff	10.2	7.1
Intraoperative increase in clarity	9.2	29.6
No light perception at times	7.1	26.5
No light perception at all during surgery	38.8	0

More than half of ophthalmologists believe that retained visual sensations could be frightening to patients and 50–80% of them think that appropriate preoperative counselling can alleviate this fear (see Table 20.7). However, only 11.4–57% offer this preoperative counselling to their patients routinely.

Table 20.7 Proportion of healthcare professionals who are aware of visual sensations during cataract surgery under local anaesthesia (%)

Visual sensation	Ophthalmologists	Anaesthesia providers	Optometry students
No light	4.6–54	33–53.6	26.4–38.9
Light	94–97.7	82.7–86	68.5–78.3
Movements	87–96	76–80.4	69.8–77.5
Flashes	77.3–86	76.5–82.1	72.9–77.5
One or more colours	93–97	78.2–81.6	63.9–70.4
Instruments	61–81	44.7–58.7	51.2–59.3
Surgeon's hand/fingers	53–65	44.7–59.2	51.2–64.8
Surgeon/medical staff	43–51	36.3–53.1	47.3–58.3
Change in light brightness	88–95	76.5–78.8	64.8–70.4

Measures to reduce the negative impact of retained visual sensations

Since retained visual sensations during ophthalmic surgery can cause fear and anxiety as well as adversely affect patient satisfaction, any intervention that can reduce its negative impact is desirable. Potentially there are several approaches.

Preoperative counselling

If patients who have not been forewarned encounter varied visual sensations during the surgery, they are unable to interpret these images and are unsure if their experience is 'normal'. For instance, patients who see vivid images may deduce that they have not been given sufficient anaesthesia. Preoperative counselling to educate patients what to expect and reassure them that these experiences are not unusual helps to allay anxiety during surgery. There are two main approaches:

Verbally advising patients specifically what to expect

Cataract patients who received preoperative counselling had a statistically significant reduction in the mean fear score compared to those who were not counselled. The effect of counselling on fear was statistically significant even after controlling for sex, age, and irrespective of first or second cataract surgery.

Showing an artist's impression

Some surgeons have used picture illustrations of visual images to counsel patients preoperatively about potential retained visual sensations during surgery. Around 20% of patients grade the value of having seen the drawings as 'very useful' while another 30% find them 'quite useful'.

Reducing the ability of patients to see during surgery

If the ability of patients to see during cataract surgery is reduced, the potential undesirable effects of these visual experiences on patients can be minimized. Judicious use of systemic sedation and administration of LA is the key.

Sedation

Oral or intravenous sedation reduces the alertness of a patient to their environment, including his visual environment. This reduced visual awareness coupled with the anxiolytic properties of the drug itself, are likely to reduce anxiety from the visual experience.

Regional anaesthetic technique

Most patients experience no light perception when given RA compared with topical anaesthesia.

Conclusion

Retained visual sensation during ophthalmic surgeries is a well-documented phenomenon that can be a source of apprehension. This can negatively impact patients' safety and satisfaction with surgery. The importance of awareness of retained visual sensations and measures to alleviate their negative impact has been reviewed in this chapter.

Key reading

Au Eong KG, Lee HM, Lim ATH, Voon LW, Yong VSH. Subjective visual experience during extracapsular cataract extraction and intraocular lens implantation under retrobulbar anaesthesia. *Eye*. 1999; 13(Pt 3a): 325–8.

Au Eong KG, Lim TH, Lee HM, Yong VSH. Subjective visual experience during phacoemulsification and intraocular lens implantation using retrobulbar anaesthesia. *J. Cataract Refract. Surg*. 2000; 26(6): 842–6.

Au Eong KG, Low CH, Heng WJ, Aung T, Lim TH, Ho SH, Yong VSH. Subjective visual experience during phacoemulsification and intraocular lens implantation under topical anaesthesia. *Ophthalmology*. 2000; 107(2): 248–50.

Laude A, Au Eong KG, Mills KB. Knowledge of visual experience during cataract surgery under anaesthesia: a nationwide survey of UK ophthalmologists. *Br. J. Ophthalmol*. 2009; 93(4): 510–12.

Rengaraj V, Radhakrishnan M, Au Eong KG, Saw SM, Srinivasan A, Mathew J, Ramasamy K, Prajna NV. Visual experience during phacoemulsification under topical versus retrobulbar anaesthesia: results of a prospective, randomised controlled trial. *Am. J. Ophthalmol*. 2004; 138(5): 782–87.

Riad W, Tan CSH, Kumar CM, Au Eong KG. What can patients see during glaucoma filtration surgery under peribulbar anaesthesia? *J. Glaucoma*. 2006; 15(5): 462–5.

Tan CSH, Au Eong KG, Kumar CM. Visual experiences during cataract surgery: what anaesthesia providers should know. *Eur. J. Anaesthesiol*. 2005; 22(6): 413–19.

Tan CSH, Au Eong KG, Lee HM (2007). Visual experiences during different stages of LASIK: Zyoptix XP microkeratome vs Intralase femtosecond laser. *Am. J. Ophthalmol*. 2007; 143(1): 90–6.

Tan CSH, Kumar CM, Fanning GL, Lai YC, Au Eong KG. A survey on the knowledge and attitudes of anaesthesia providers in the United States of America, United Kingdom and Singapore on visual experiences during cataract surgery. *Eur. J. Anaesthesiol*. 2006; 23(4): 276–81.

Tan CSH, Mahmood U, O'Brien PD, Beatty S, Kwok AKH, Lee VYW, Au Eong KG. Visual experiences during vitreous surgery under regional anaesthesia: a multicentre study. *Am. J. Ophthalmol*. 2005; 140(6): 971–5.

Voon LW, Au Eong KG, Saw SM, Verma D, Laude A. Effect of preoperative counselling on patient fear from the visual experience during phacoemulsification under topical anaesthesia: multicentre randomised clinical trial. *J. Cataract Refract. Surg*. 2005; 31(10): 1966–9.

Chapter 21

Complications of ophthalmic regional anaesthesia

Professor Chandra M. Kumar

Introduction

Selection of anaesthesia technique varies widely worldwide. Ophthalmic RA is most commonly employed for routine surgical procedures. These are performed by injecting LA through a needle or blunt cannula. Needle-based blocks (intraconal or retrobulbar and extraconal or peribulbar) have been the traditional method to achieve anaesthesia. In recent years, cannula-based blocks (sub-Tenon's) have become more popular in many countries. Topical anaesthesia for selected patients undergoing simple procedures may be associated with inadequate analgesia, pain and discomfort, gross patient movement, and poor operating conditions.

- The choice of anaesthesia technique depends on many factors including:
  - Surgical procedure
  - Duration
  - Surgeon's preference
  - Patient's medical condition
  - Patient preference
  - Available resources
- Safety of orbital blocks depends on:
  - Knowledge of anatomy
  - Understanding the relationship between the globe and orbit
  - Ophthalmologic background of the patient
  - Gaze of the eye during the injection
  - Selection of equipment
  - LA agent utilized
  - Adjuvant used
- Despite the increased awareness and knowledge, complications continue to be reported. This chapter deals with sight- and life-threatening complications which may follow from the use of needle- and cannula-based orbital blocks (see Tables 21.1 & 21.2). Complications may be simple or serious, local or systemic, immediate or late.
  Complications also occur from injected drugs such as LA agent or adjuvant.

Table 21.1 Major complications of needle blocks (modified from Kumar and Dowd 2006)

Complications	Mechanism	Risk factors	Incidence	Prevention	Treatment
Inadvertent subarachnoid anaesthesia (brainstem anaesthesia)	Subject to debate but spread through optic nerve sheath or through the orbital foramina	Placement of long needle into the apex	0.3–0.8% (retrobulbar) Unknown (peribulbar)	Avoid using long needle	Extensive cardiorespiratory support
Ocular perforation	Direct needle entry into the globe through sclera	Placement of needle angled towards the apex	3:4000 (retrobulbar block) 1:16224 (peribulbar block)	Attention to anatomy and appropriate technique	Immediate ophthalmic opinion
Retrobulbar haemorrhage	Damage to arterial or venous blood vessels behind the globe	Elderly, receiving steroids, NSAID, aspirin	0.1–3%	Limit insertion of needle <31mm in the relatively avascular area	Immediate oculocompression, ophthalmic opinion and decompression surgery if necessary
Globe ischaemia	Interruption of blood flow	Prolonged oculocompression	Unknown	Use pressure-limiting oculocompression device	Ophthalmic opinion
Optic nerve atrophy	Direct damage to nerve, central retinal artery or secondary to haemorrhage		Unknown	Careful needle placement	Ophthalmic opinion

(continued)

Table 21.1 (Contd.)

Complications	Mechanism	Risk factors	Incidence	Prevention	Treatment
Damage to the motor nerve of the inferior rectus and inferior oblique muscles	Direct trauma to the nerve	Insertion of needle at the junction of medial 2/3rd and lateral 1/3rd of inferior orbital margin	Unknown	Careful needle placement avoiding the nerve	Ophthalmic opinion
Prolonged extra-ocular muscle malfunction	Prolonged exposure of fine muscle fibres, injection of local anaesthetic agent into the muscle	May be associated with non-use of hyaluronidase	Unknown	Proper placement of needle	Ophthalmic opinion
Orbital swelling	Infection Excessive dose of hyaluronidase	Poor technique	Unknown	Aseptic technique Use of recommended dose of hyaluronidase	Antibiotics, steroids, ophthalmic opinion

Table 21.2 Limitations and relative contraindications of sub-Tenon's block (modified from Kumar and Dodds 2006)

Limitations
Previous sub-Tenon's block in the same quadrant
Previous extensive vitreoretinal surgery
Previous repeated strabismus surgery
Eye trauma
Infection to the orbit
Relative contraindications
Severe ocular pemphigoid
Surgery requiring complete akinesia (viscacanalstomy)
Surgery where chemosis and subconjunctival haemorrhage may compromise the outcome of surgery (glaucoma filtration surgery)

Table 21.3 Sight- and life-threatening complications of sub-Tenon's block

Complications	Possible mechanism	Risk factors	Incidence	Prevention	Treatment
Brainstem anaesthesia	Injection into the optic nerve sheath Unintentional perforation of Tenon's capsule and spread of LA to CNS through one of the orbital foramen	Deep posterior injection	Unknown	Adhere to basic anatomy, use shorter sub-Tenon's cannulae	Extensive cardiorespiratory support
Globe penetration	Improper dissection	Inexperienced user, poor technique, previous surgery	Unknown	Careful use of technique and adhere to basic anatomy	Immediate senior ophthalmic opinion
Intraorbital, orbital and/or retrobulbar haemorrhage	Trauma to blood vessel Rupture of sclerotic blood vessel	Patients receiving aspirin or clopidogrel Inappropriate technique	Unknown	Adhere to anatomy	Immediate oculocompression, ophthalmologic opinion and decompression surgery
Retinal ischaemia	Increase in IOP Retrobulbar haemorrhage Compression of blood vessel	High volume of LA Glaucoma Compromised circulation to retinal artery	Unknown	Void deep posterior injection	Ophthalmic opinion

Optic nerve damage	Direct trauma Optic neuropathy	Posterior injection High concentration of LA	Unknown	Avoid deep posterior injection, use recommended dose of appropriate LA	Ophthalmic opinion
Rectus muscle dysfunction	Direct trauma to muscle Injection of LA into the muscle Prolonged exposure of rectus muscle fibres with LA agent	Not known	Unknown	Proper placement of cannula Adhere to anatomy Avoid forceful injection	Ophthalmic opinion
Orbital swelling	Infection Excessive dose of hyaluronidase	Poor technique	Unknown	Aseptic technique, use recommended dose of hyaluronidase	Antibiotics, steroids and ophthalmic opinion

Pain during injection

Patients may be anxious prior to and during ophthalmic surgery. This is due to anticipated pain, discomfort, or fear of seeing something during surgery. Untreated pain and anxiety can lead to poor patient and surgeon satisfaction.

- All LA eye drops sting on application. Proxymetacaine 0.5% and oxybuprocaine 0.4% eye drops provide inadequate surface anaesthesia whilst tetracaine 1% provides good surface anaesthesia
- There are disagreements about the superiority of an individual RA technique. The incidence of pain following needle- or cannula-based blocks varies widely from paper to paper. In one study, sub-Tenon's block caused pain on injection in 43% of patients:
  - Varied between visual analogue scale (VAS) 1–3: 0—no pain, 10—very severe pain
- Pain during sub-Tenon's block may occur due to stretching of the potential sub-Tenon's space especially with long metal posterior sub-Tenon's cannulae. Smaller flexible cannulae appear to offer benefit
- All concentrated LA agents cause burning sensation or pain during injection:
  - The incidence of pain can be reduced by reassurance and slow injection of warm LA agent
  - Injection of a diluted LA agent (0.01%) before the main concentrated injection during needle block also reduces discomfort

Chemosis

Chemosis refers to the swelling of conjunctiva caused by anterior spread of the injected LA agent. The incidence of chemosis varies with the technique used and the volume of injected LA.

- Needle-based blocks:
  - The incidence of chemosis is more localized and much rarer (<2%)
  - The injected LA spreads anteriorly because of the density of tissue in the intraconal compartment and the physics of fluid taking the path of least resistance
  - There is no distinct anatomical separation between the extraconal and intraconal compartments (see 📖 Injections and spread of local anaesthetic agents, pp. 32–33) so chemosis can occur with either type of block
  - Injection of higher volumes of LA increases the likelihood of chemosis
- Cannula-based blocks:
  - On the other hand the incidence of chemosis after sub-Tenon's block is much higher and ranges anywhere from 23–100%
  - It often spreads to other quadrants in addition to the quadrant injected
  - Chemosis during sub-Tenon's block occurs when the Tenon's capsule is improperly dissected
  - Higher volumes of LA are associated with more chemosis
  - Short or ultra-short sub-Tenon's cannulae produce the greatest degree of chemosis.

Chemosis may resolve with time spontaneously or with the application of locally applied orbital pressure and generally does not interfere with the surgery.

Orbital haemorrhage

Sub-conjunctival haemorrhage

Damage to small superficial vessels can be inflicted by the needle or scissors during the dissection of Tenon's capsule. This is manifested as sub-conjunctival haemorrhage, bruising or simple redness and may be associated with the lid ecchymosis.

- The incidence of sub-conjunctival haemorrhage varies from 1–2.75% following needle-based blocks
- The sub-Tenon's block has a much higher incidence of subconjunctival haemorrhage, ranging from 23–46%. This further increases to 100% with shorter cannulae
- Occurs more commonly in elderly patients especially those taking steroids, NSAIDs or aspirin:
  - According to a recent report, subconjunctival haemorrhage occurred in 19% in the control group, 40% in the clopidogrel group, 35% in the warfarin group and 21% in the aspirin group
- Sub-conjunctival haemorrhage can be reduced by careful dissection, application of topical epinephrine or (controversially) with the use of hand-held cautery
- Sub-conjunctival haemorrhage usually resolves within a few days

Retrobulbar/orbital haemorrhage

Retrobulbar haemorrhage occurs due to damage of either venous or arterial vessels in the posterior part of the orbit.

- Venous bleeding is slow and usually resolves with pressure and time:
  - Often no sequellae and surgery proceeds as planned
- Arterial bleeding is rapid and manifested by increasing proptosis, sub-conjunctival and peri-orbital haemorrhage and a dramatic increase in intra-ocular pressure
- Deep placement of a long needle into the orbital apex or superior orbit can lead to retrobulbar haemorrhage. Vortex vein bleeding has been reported with sub-Tenon's block using long metallic cannula
- It is more likely to occur in elderly patients receiving steroids, aspirin, NSAIDs, and anti-coagulants
- The incidence of retrobulbar haemorrhage varies from 0.44 to 3% with needle-based blocks
- The incidence of orbital and retrobulbar haemorrhage is rare, but has been reported, with posterior sub-Tenon's block
- A retrobulbar haemorrhage should be suspected when the conjunctiva is diffusely erythematous and the eye is proptotic (bulging forward)
- Intra-ocular pressure should be determined and retinal circulation should be checked
- Treatment is directed towards reducing intra-ocular pressure and minimising its effects on the retinal circulation
- Immediate oculocompression should be considered. If the condition is sight-threatening, urgent surgical decompression may be required
- Ophthalmologists should be consulted to evaluate the degree of haemorrhage and review the need for an urgent lateral canthotomy

- Lateral canthotomy is an incision performed at the lateral canthus in order to allow the lids greater separation, promoting forward movement of orbital contents and relief of pressure induced by a rapidly expanding arterial based retrobulbar haemorrhage (see Figure 21.1)
- Minimize risk of retrobulbar haemorrhage by:
  - Allaying patient anxiety. The blood vessels behind the eye become engorged in anxious patients due to straining and are readily punctured. The anxious, straining patient may need some sedation and should be encouraged to breathe quietly through an open mouth
  - The number of injections into the orbit should be limited hence creating less chance of damaging a blood vessel
  - Fine needles may be less traumatic than thicker ones
  - The injection should be limited to the inferotemporal quadrant and medial canthal area which are relatively avascular hence less hazardous
  - Firm digital pressure may be applied to the orbit as soon as the needle is withdrawn after any injection, as this reduces any tendency to bleed

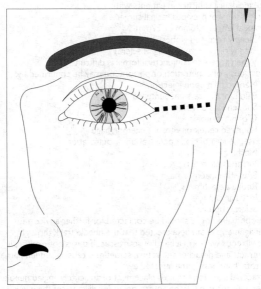

Fig. 21.1 Lateral canthotomy: emergent procedure to relieve orbital compartment pressure. After prep, local anaesthetic is infiltrated from the lateral canthus in temporal direction. A haemostat is then applied along the indicated line to devascularize the tissue prior to cutting the canthal tendon. (Reprinted with permission from: Au Eong KG (2002). 6th Yahya Cohen Lecture: Visual experience during cataract surgery. *Ann Acad Med Singapore*, **31**(5):666–74).

Globe penetration and perforation

The sclera is a tough tissue that provides structural rigidity to the globe. It is typically not perforated easily.

- Globe penetration/perforation has been reported following:
  - Intraconal block
  - Extraconal injection
  - Sub-Tenon's block
  - Even following infiltration for more minor procedures such as eyelid surgery
- Classification
  - Penetration:
    — Is defined as a single entrance lesion through the globe's sclera
  - Perforation:
    — Is a through and through, double-puncture injury
    — Both entry and exit wounds through the sclera are present
- Perforations tend to be more severe, particularly if multiple entry and exit wounds are present.
- The incidence varies from 0.1 in 12,000 (retrobulbar) and 1 in 16,224 (peribulbar) and is rare with sub-Tenon's block
- The incidence is higher in patients with:
  - A history of previous retinal surgery
  - Axial length >26mm or 27mm
  - Deeply recessed globes
  - Staphyloma (outpouching of sclera)
  - When access to conjunctival fornix is difficult
- A diagnosis of penetration or perforation may be confirmed by:
  - Marked pain upon injection
  - Pain is not always encountered
  - Sudden loss of vision
  - Globe hypotonia
  - Poor red reflex or vitreous haemorrhage
- Consequences of globe penetration or perforation:
  - Nothing
  - Vitreous haemorrhage
  - Subretinal haemorrhage
  - Retina detachment
  - Macular damage
  - Scleral rupture
- An ophthalmologist should be contacted for further advice and management. It can be expected that the needle track through the vitreous will form a band of scar tissue. If this is not excised, it contracts and detaches the retina, sometimes causing sudden partial or total blindness in the affected eye
- Intraconal injection requires placement of an acutely angled needle deep into the orbit. If the antero-posterior distance of the eye is significantly longer than average, there is a greater risk of accidental injection into the posterior part of the globe by a steeply angulated needle

- Antero-posterior length is increased with:
  - Myopia
  - Staphyloma (aberrant outpouched section of globe)
  - An *in-situ* scleral buckle deforming the globe, enlarging the axial length
- ❶ Minimize risk of penetrating or perforating injury by:
  - Being aware that globes differ in length and shape
  - Noting the relationship between the globe and orbit. A deeply recessed globe is at greater risk if the needle is acutely angled
  - Ideally, confirmation of globe length/shape via a preoperative ultrasound if the eye is suspected to be myopic (longer than typical)
  - In most patients who present for cataract surgery an ultrasound measure (biometry) of the globe's axial length is obtained by the ophthalmologist in order to calculate the power of the required intra-ocular lens
  - Normal globes have an axial length of 20–24mm
  - High myopes may have much longer axial lengths (>26mm) and extreme caution should be exercised in these patients
  - High myopes may have thin sclera that can be injured by sub-Tenon's cannula or scissors
  - Presence of *in-situ* scleral buckle may increase antero-posterior length of the globe
  - The axial length in patients undergoing glaucoma, retina, or strabismus surgery is not usually measured
  - Staphaloma may be noted on ultrasound exam
- Additionally, the surface anatomy should be assessed to determine the globe–orbit relationship
  - A recessed globe is at greater risk of posterior pole injury
  - The extraconal approach of shallower needle placement with minimal angulation may diminish the likelihood of encountering the globe's hind surface
  - However, inadvertent needle penetration can nonetheless occur at the globe's periphery
- Patients presenting with repeated VR surgery may have anatomy distorted by an *in-situ* sclera buckle
- Knowledge of orbital anatomy and axial length, use of a technique based on sound principles, shallow placement of a short needle tangential to the globe, and the use of non-metallic sub-Tenon's cannulae may reduce this complication

Nerve damage

Optic nerve injury

This complication is exceedingly rare. It is usually associated with use of a long needle, inserted deeply and directed towards the apex of the orbit.

- It may result in:
  - Visual field loss
  - Blindness
  - Central retinal artery occlusion
  - Orbital epidural
  - Brainstem anaesthesia
- Optic nerve damage may result from:
  - Direct placement of the needle into the nerve
  - A long rigid sub-Tenon's cannula
  - Deep placement of sub-Tenon's scissors
  - Injection of LA into the nerve sheath leading to compression
  - Ischaemia secondary to vascular occlusion following vasoconstriction of blood vessels with epinephrine containing LA solution
  - Obstruction of the central retinal artery:
    — This is the first and smallest branch of the ophthalmic artery
    — It runs for a short distance within the dural sheath of the optic nerve and about 35mm from the orbital margin, pierces the nerve advancing forward in the centre of the nerve to the retina
    — Damage to the artery may cause bleeding into the confined space of the optic nerve sheath, compressing and obstructing blood flow
    — If the complication is recognized soon enough, it may be possible to perform surgical decompression of the optic nerve
- ❶ Minimize risk: damage to the optic nerve can be avoided by:
  - Appreciating the orbital anatomy
  - Appropriate needle placement—avoid apical direction
  - Use of needle <31mm in length
  - Maintaining the eye in neutral gaze position—the practice of having the patient look upwards and inward brings the optic nerve directly into the path of an infero-temporally placed needle

Optic nerve atrophy

This is a delayed, extremely rare complication which may lead to partial or complete visual loss.

- Optic atrophy and retinal vascular occlusion may be caused by:
  - Direct damage to the optic nerve
  - Injection into the optic nerve sheath
  - Haemorrhage within the nerve sheath with or without acute retinal vascular occlusion
  - Central retinal artery obstruction, following severe retrobulbar haemorrhage
- The mechanism is not very clear but may involve shutdown of optic nerve retinal microvasculature

- There is no evidence to suggest that epinephrine in standard vasoconstrictor concentration is causative
- ❶ Minimize risk by:
  - Careful needle placement avoiding the optic nerve (see 📖 Gaze position, p. 99)
  - Avoiding injection of LA when resistance to injection is noted

Damage to the motor nerve of inferior rectus and oblique muscles

- Another very rare complication which may occur when a needle is introduced through the skin at the junction point at the medial 2/3rd and lateral 1/3rd position along the inferior orbital rim
- Nerve damage usually occurs following direct trauma to the nerve during injection
- This complication may be avoided by introducing a needle into the infero-temporal quadrant further laterally

Globe ischaemia

A mechanical orbital decompression device is commonly used to promote ocular hypotony ('soften the eye'). It is possible for these devices to induce globe ischaemia.

- Blood flow to the retina, choroids and optic nerve depends on the balance between intra-ocular pressure and the mean local arterial blood pressure
- The externally applied pressure has the potential to significantly reduce blood flow to these vital areas
- This may occur especially in the presence of significant local arterial disease, orbital haemorrhage or increased intra-ocular pressure
- Patients with scleroderma have a markedly limited orbital capacity for injected local anaesthetic agent
- ❶ Minimize risk of globe ischaemia by:
  - Careful history-taking
  - Noting presence of glaucoma
  - Limiting anaesthetic agent and avoid high-volume injection
  - The use of non-epinephrine-containing solution

Prolonged extra-ocular muscle malfunction

Prolonged extra-ocular muscle malfunction presents as diplopia and ptosis often 24–48h postoperatively. It frequently resolves spontaneously; however, if persistent, corrective lenses or surgery may be indicated.

- Possible causes of postoperative extra-ocular muscle dysfunction include:
  - Local anaesthetic myotoxicity
  - Direct muscle injury
  - Motor nerve injury
  - Vascular injury
- The inadvertent injection of a LA agent into any extra-ocular muscle body may result in prolonged weakness, fibrosis or even necrosis of the muscle. Other possibilities include prolonged exposure of thin rectus muscle fibres with highly concentrated LA agent and damage to the motor nerve supplying the muscle.
- A more lateral infero temporal approach than the traditionally described 1/3rd and 2/3rd junction point at the inferior orbital rim places the needle between the lateral and inferior rectus muscles and is a more suitable site for injections.
- Evidence suggests that the addition of hyaluronidase to the LA agent helps disperse the solution.
- Highest incidence associated with use of 0.75% bupivacaine.
- Persistent diplopia following LA may warrant referral to a squint surgeon as surgical intervention to the affected muscle may be required. If there is no nerve damage, function normally returns in 2–3 weeks. If recovery is delayed for more than 6 weeks, there is a 25% chance of permanent damage.
- ❶ Minimize risk of postoperative strabismus:
  - Thorough knowledge of three-dimensional anatomy of the orbit
  - Proper placement of needle thus avoiding muscle and nerves
  - Avoid 0.75% bupivacaine
  - Appropriate use of LA agent volume

Complications of facial nerve block

Facial nerve block is performed to block orbicularis oculi muscle and attenuate lid squeezing (see 📖 Facial nerve block, p. 102). The low-volume classical retrobulbar block technique does not affect the facial nerve. The nerve may be blocked at several points after exiting from the base of the skull.

- Complications include:
  - Pain on injection
  - Bruising of eyelids or face
  - Transient hemifacial palsy
  - Spread of LA to the vagus nerve, glossopharyngeal or spinal accessory nerves
  - Neurogenic pulmonary oedema
  - Other rare reported complications
- More recently advocated needle-block techniques utilizing higher-volume local anaesthetic usually block the terminal branches of the 7th cranial nerve. Paralysis of orbicularis is often not required during modern phacoemulsification surgery.

Central nervous system spread and brainstem anaesthesia

Spread of LA agent into the central nervous system has been reported after needle-based as well as cannula-based blocks.

- The cerebral dura mater provides a tubular sheath for the optic nerve as it passes through the optic foramen and is a potential conduit for LA to pass subdurally or epidurally into the brain
- Central spread occurs if the needle tip has perforated the optic nerve sheath:
  - Puncture of the optic nerve sheath by the needle provides an entry port for LAs into the subarachnoid space
  - The mechanism of brainstem anaesthesia is subject to debate as epidural spread has also been postulated
- Even a small volume of LA agent may enter the central nervous system and/or cross the optic chiasma to the opposite eye and leading to life-threatening and sight-threatening complications
  - It has been shown radiologically that communication is possible from the subdural space of the optic nerve to the optic chiasma and subsequently to the subarachnoid space surrounding the pons and midbrain
- The signs and symptoms of central spread are varied and depend upon which part of the central nervous system is exposed to the LA agent:
  - Pons
  - Midbrain
  - Cranial nerves
- The time of onset of symptoms is variable but usually develops within the first 15min after the injection and may last 2–3h
- Unexplained onset of sensorial changes should be taken seriously
- Drowsiness, light-headedness, confusion, loss of verbal contact, cranial nerve palsies, convulsions, respiratory depression or respiratory arrest and even cardiac arrest may occur. Contralateral pupil may be areflexic and dilated
- Supportive cardiopulmonary treatment throughout the duration of effect is indicated:
  - Reassurance
  - Ventilatory support with oxygen
  - Intravenous fluid therapy
  - Pharmacological support (vagolytics, vasopressors, vasodilators or adrenergic blocking agents) may be required as dictated by close monitoring of vital signs
- Minimize risk of central spread and brainstem anaesthesia:
  - Any injection should be made with the patient looking in neutral gaze eye position
    - This keeps the optic nerve slack and out of the way of the advancing needle
    - If the needle accidently encounters the optic nerve in this gaze, it is unlikely to damage or perforate the optic nerve sheath because the looseness of the nerve allows it to be pushed aside

- • If the optic nerve is stretched and taut, the nerve cannot be easily pushed aside by the oncoming needle
- • The injection should not be made too deep into the orbit, where the optic nerve is tethered to its sheath as it emerges through the optic foramen
- • A needle <31mm is unlikely to reach that posterior into the apex of the orbit
- • If there is any resistance to injection, the needle should be withdrawn and repositioned before injection

Complications related to injectable local anaesthetic agent

The incidence of systemic toxicity with LA (see ⊞ Toxicity, pp. 60–61) depends on the site of injection, vascularity of the site, the total dose administered, specific drug used, speed of injection, use of epinephrine or other agents as an additive and other factors. The injected LA can enter the CNS (see ⊞ Central nervous system spread and brainstem anaesthesia, pp. 348–349) or systemically absorbed into the circulation.

Systemic absorption

- Injection into an orbital vessel can have systemic consequences
- Intra-arterial injection can result in retrograde arterial flow of the local anaesthetic and rapid dispersion into the cerebral circulation
- The onset of central nervous system toxicity in this case is almost instantaneous
- Convulsions may begin prior to completion of the injection
- A harbinger of more gradual absorption of LA is patient complaint of a metallic taste or tinnitus
- This may be followed by:
  - Excitement
  - Loss of consciousness
  - Frank seizures
  - Rarely by cardiovascular collapse
- Treatment:
  - Provide oxygen
  - Maintain and protect the airway
  - Seizures are treated with intravenous sedatives and/or small doses of intravenous induction agents (propofol, sodium thiopental etc).
  - Supportive cardiopulmonary treatment as indicated
- Minimize risk of intravascular injection:
  - Utilization of minimum effective dose in terms of volume and concentration
  - Consider test aspiration before injection (debatable efficacy)
  - Slow rate of injection in fractional amounts while maintaining verbal contact with the patient for reporting of possible harbinger symptoms.

Allergic reaction

- Hypersensitivity reaction is very unlikely with the amide group of LA. History of previous exposure should be sought.

Complications related to topical local anaesthetic agent

Topical local anaesthetic agents

The most common issue is stinging sensation upon instillation of drops.

Corneal effects

- Decreased tear production
- Epithelial toxicity
- Endothelial toxicity
- Microbial contamination

Systemic effects

- Cocaine may be absorbed and have cardiovascular implications including hypertension, myocardial ischemia, and others
- Allergic and idiosyncratic responses:
  - Proparacaine—contact dermatitis
- Stevens–Johnson syndrome
- Endophthalmitis (see ⚏ Disadvantages of ophthalmic topical anaesthesia, pp. 132–133)

Adverse surgical outcomes of topical anaesthesia

- Inadequate analgesia
- Pain and discomfort
- Lid squeezing and blepharospasm
- Roaming eye
- Patient inability to tolerate procedure
- Need for 'vocal local'
- Need for increased sedation which may result in possible airway obstruction, compromised ventilation, patient confusion, and/or need to induce GA (⚏ see Complications during monitored sedation, pp. 146–148)
- Abrupt gross patient movement
- Poor surgical operating conditions
- Poor visual outcome

Complications related to adjuvants

Epinephrine

- Admixture with epinephrine is commonly used to prolong the block and increase its solidity
- A concentration (1:200,000) is typically used:
  - More concentrated doses may be associated with local ischaemia, impaired perfusion, and systemic side effects
- Consider avoiding epinephrine in the presence of arterial disease

Hyaluronidase

- Hyaluronidase has been shown to improve the effectiveness and the quality of needle-based blocks but its role in sub-Tenon's block is controversial
- The incidence of muscle dysfunction (postoperative strabismus) may be higher in the absence of hyaluronidase
- The amount of hyaluronidase used varies from 5–1500IU:
  - 15IU/ml is the recommended and commonly used effective concentration
- Rare allergic reaction, orbital pseudotumour and orbital swelling have been reported
- Some formulations contain thimerosal
- May be of bovine, ovine, or recombinant DNA origin

Conclusion

Although complications of orbital blocks are rare, they can occur and no technique is absolutely safe. Sound knowledge of orbital anatomy, ophthalmic physiology, and pharmacology of the anaesthesia and ophthalmic drugs are prerequisites before embarking on orbital RA. This should be augmented by training in techniques obtained in clinical settings from practitioners with broad experience and knowledge.

Key reading

Hamilton RC. A discourse on the complications of retrobulbar and perbulbar blockade. *Can. J. Ophthalmol.* 2000; 35: 363–72.

Kumar C, Dowd T. Ophthalmic regional anaesthesia. *Curr. Opin. Anaesthesiol.* 2008; 21: 632–7.

Kumar CM, Dodds C. Sub-Tenon's anesthesia. *Ophthalmol. Clin. North Am.* 2006; 19: 209–19.

Kumar CM, Dowd TC. Complications of ophthalmic regional blocks: their treatment and prevention. *Ophthalmologica.* 2006; 220: 73–82.

Kumar CM. Needle-based blocks for 21st-century ophthalmology. *Acta. Ophthalmol.* 2010; Epub ahead of print.

Rubin AP. Complications of local anaesthesia for ophthalmic surgery. *British J. Anaesthesia.* 1995; 75: 93–96.

Chapter 22

Patient positioning for eye surgery

Mr Tom Eke

Dr Howard Palte

Introduction

Positioning of the patient is be dictated by the type of operation proposed, the type of anaesthesia needed, the requirements of the surgeon (surgical access and ease), and the comfort of the patient. Supine position is standard. Traditionally, eye surgery has used a flat bed or trolley, but reclining surgical chairs (evolved from traditional 'dentist's chairs') are now common.

Standard positioning

General

- Supine position is standard for easy access for surgeon and anaesthetist
- Position the patient optimally beneath operating microscope
- Pad pressure points—especially elbows/heels (see Figure 22.1)
- Consider peripheral nerve injury mechanisms
- Compression/stretching/ischaemia
- Most patients are happier if they sit up a little
- Chair back at 10–20° above horizontal
- Anaesthetist situated at patient's side
- Patients instructed to squeeze anaesthetist's or nurse's hand if they have any concerns or pain during surgery. Hand-holding assists in active monitoring of the patient (see Figure 22.1)

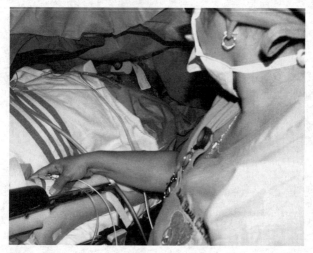

Fig. 22.1 Tenting of surgical drape. Note position of anaesthetist and use of chin-tilt device.

Head

- Headrest flat so that face points to overhead microscope
- Soft pad/gel support under head—prevents pressure alopecia
- Tape securely for steady position
- Avoid substantial flexion/extension of neck
- Non-operative eye should be protected
- For general anaesthesia patients one must protect the nonoperative eye from drying and injury, especially corneal abrasion. Use tape/eyepad/eyeshield (see Figure 22.2).
- Secure nasal oxygen cannula—avoid displacement

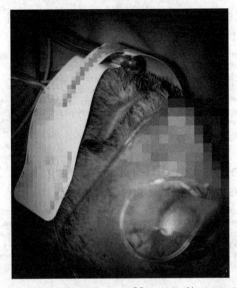

Fig. 22.2 Accessory equipment to attenuate CO_2 retention. Note protective shield on non-operative eye.

Limbs

- Pillows under knees for lumbar support
- Limit the Trendelenburg tilt—consider use of non-sliding mattress
- Secure arms at sides to prevent unexpected hand movement towards the operative field (see Figure 22.1)
- Safety straps to prevent accidental falls

Anaesthetic considerations

- Insert IV cannula and pulse oximeter probe on the side closest to the anaesthetist for ready access
- Elevate and fix drapes away from patient's face (see Figure 22.1)
  - Permits direct vision of patient
  - Attenuates claustrophobia issues
- Anaesthetist or nurse monitoring the patient sits on low chair and looks up towards patient and holds the hand of the patient
- Consider use of patient warming convection device in elderly patients for longer procedures

Procedures requiring non-standard positioning

Non-standard positioning of patient may be required under the following situations:
- Removal of object from anterior chamber (e.g. foreign body) when supine position risks object falling more posteriorly
- Upright positioning may be helpful when gas bubble used as part of retinal detachment correction. Prone surgery (floating bubble) now superseded by heavy liquid use
- Upright position may help in some cases

Patient's conditions requiring non-standard positioning

Many medical conditions will prevent a patient from lying flat and supine for surgery. Some patients may have several minor problems, which combine to prevent normal positioning. Common examples include orthopnoea due to cardiac failure, chronic obstructive pulmonary disease (COPD) or motor neuronal disease; spinal deformity (kyphosis: osteoporosis, ankylosing spondylitis), obesity and others.

Positioning strategies for non-standard cases

The following strategies can be considered if a patient cannot lie flat:
- Adjust the patient's chair
  Sit patient more upright, recline head back
  Sit patient up, then use Trendelenburg (recline) position
  Trendelenburg in supine patient
- Change the patient's chair
  A different model may have different positions
  Orthopedic tables may have big range of tilt
  May need bespoke adjustment of chair/table in extreme cases
- Re-position the surgeon
  Surgeon may need to stand instead of sit
  Surgeon may need a seat that is higher/lower/more mobile
  Temporal or nasal approach
  Face-to-face approach
- Move the position of the microscope
  Temporal or nasal approach instead of superior
  Rotate the microscope away from vertical
- General anaesthesia instead of MAC may be useful in certain cases
- Change the RA technique
  Topical anaesthesia retains eye movement, keeps eye 'on axis'

- Change the operation
  E.g. laser instead of trabeculectomy for glaucoma
- Postpone the operation
  Reschedule and then re-evaluate elective cases once patient in more
  optimal condition

Extreme positioning strategies

Patient cannot lie flat, but can extend neck (Figure 22.3)
- E.g. severe orthopnoea
- Standing temporal approach for phacoemulsification etc.:
  - Operating chair more upright
  - Headrest horizontal (facing overhead microscope)
  - Local anaesthesia
  - Surgeon may have to stand instead of sit
  - Temporal incision may be easier for phacoemulsification
  - Raise fluid bottles, as eye is higher than usual

Patient can lie flat, but has fixed neck flexion (Figure 22.4)
- E.g. ankylosing spondylitis, otherwise healthy
- Extreme Trendelburg positioning for phacoemulsification, etc.:
  - Orthopaedic tilting table or parachute-like harness
  - Need to ensure patient is secure and will not fall

Patient cannot lie flat and can not extend neck (Figure 22.5)
- E.g. severe orthopnoea with stiff neck
- Face-to-face positioning for phacoemulsification, etc.:
  - Patient seated, chair/head reclined as much as possible
  - Surgeon faces patient (standing or sitting)
  - Microscope rotated toward horizontal
  - Inferior corneal incision for phacoemulsification
  - Topical anaesthesia ensures eye is 'on axis' for phacoemulsification
  - Raise fluid bottles, as eye is higher than usual
  - Needs experienced surgeon
  - Can be used for any patient, no additional equipment needed

For complex cases, patient, surgeon, and anaesthetist must be happy with positioning before surgery commences

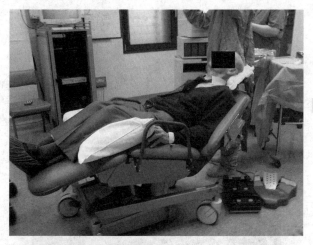

Fig. 22.3 Patient cannot lie flat, but can extend neck.

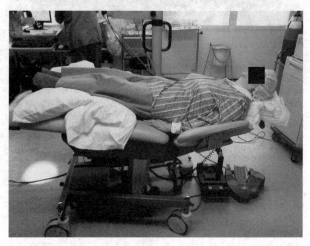

Fig. 22.4 Pateint can lie flat, but has fixed neck flexion.

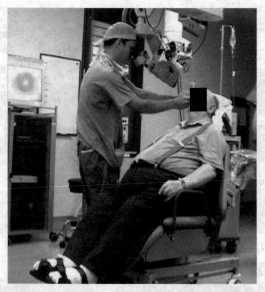

Fig. 22.5 Patient cannot lie flat and cannot extend neck.

Postoperative postures after VR surgery

Following VR surgery patients may need to positioned in a particular posture to ensure that the gas bubble in the eye is in the optimal position. When the retinal break is superior the optimal position is sitting upright and if the hole is posterior the optimal position is face down. Patients are able to posture immediately after surgery if RA has been used. If GA is used then the patient will have to recover sufficiently before they are able to adopt the optimal position.

Specific anaesthesia issues

CO_2 retention
- May manifest as anxiety, tachycardia, hypertension, sweating etc. Elevated baseline CO_2 (if monitored) may be seen on the capnograph
- Surgical drape tightly adherent to face
- Prevention by removal of retained CO_2 from environment:
  - Elevate surgical drape away from face (see Figure 22.1).
  - Blow air under drapes
  - Suction catheter on chin or nasal 'tent' (see Figure 22.2)

Obstructive sleep apnoea (OSA)
- Common problem associated with obesity—manifests with hypoxia/hypercarbia
- Curtail use of sedatives (especially narcotics)
- Chin tilt device may be of benefit (see Figure 22.1)
- Obesity—requirement for additional padding of pressure points

General anaesthetic technique
- Position ETT/LMA away from nose/upper face (see Figure 22.6)
- Tape securely to avoid movement/dislodgement (see Figure 22.6)
- CO_2 line in lateral position—circumvents obstruction by surgical drape (see Figure 22.6)
- Neck position—neutral may need to use accessory neck roll (see Figure 22.6)
- Avoid head compression against surgical ring support
- Consider haemodynamic/respiratory changes associated with GA

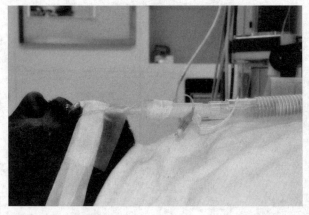

Fig. 22.6 GA-securing ETT away from operative field. Note neutral position neck and lateral position capnography line.

Deep vein thrombosis (DVT)
- Risk with prolonged surgery (>2–3h)
- Especially oculoplastic/reconstruction/trauma cases
- Consider use of intermittent or sequential calf-compression device/ compression stockings

Conclusion

Positioning of the patient on the operating table is dictated by the type of operation proposed, the type of anaesthesia, the requirements of the surgeon (surgical access and ease) and the comfort of the patient. Patients can be positioned appropriately and surgeons can also adopt other positions in conditions and situations which otherwise do not allow standard supine flat position.

Key reading

Rogers GM, Goins KM. Cataract surgery in the patient that cannot lie flat. *Curr. Opin. Ophthalmol.* 2010; 21: 71–4.

Chapter 23

Postoperative management

Dr Irina Gasanova

Dr Girish Joshi

Introduction

In recent years, there has been a significant increase in the number of ophthalmic surgical procedures performed due to an ageing population and an increase in patients with multiple comorbidities such as hypertension and diabetes. With improved surgical techniques, many routine ophthalmic procedures can now be performed using local/regional anaesthesia techniques with minimal sedation, with only a few requiring general anaesthesia (GA). Also, an increasing number of ophthalmic procedures are performed on an outpatient basis. The perioperative outcome after an ophthalmic procedure performed on outpatient basis is similar to that performed on an inpatient basis. Importantly, the level of postoperative care in outpatients should be similar to inpatients. The goal of postoperative care is to optimize the outcome of surgery through early recognition and management of complications of anaesthesia and surgery. This chapter will review the postoperative management of an adult patient undergoing ophthalmic surgery.

Procedures that can be performed under local/regional anaesthesia:
- Eyelid surgery
- Blepharoplasty
- Tarsoplasty
- Chalazion operations
- Trabeculectomy
- Strabismus correction
- Cataract surgery
- Vitreoretinal surgery
- Cryopexy and laser surgery
- Operations on the lacrimal apparatus

Situations and procedures that may require GA:
- Examination under anaesthesia
- Patients who refuse the operation under LA
- Patients with claustrophobia
- Patients with learning disabilities/movement disorder, dementia
- Patients unable to lie flat and remain motionless
- Extensive surgical procedures (e.g., oculoplasty, dacrocystorhinostomy, and traumatic eye injury)

Benefits of local/regional anaesthesia techniques include:
- Maintain patient alertness
- Reduce the incidence of postoperative pain, nausea and vomiting
- Avoid adverse effects associated with GA
- Facilitate recovery and improve patient satisfaction

Benefits of ophthalmic surgery performed on an outpatient basis:
- Reduce disruption to the patient's normal activity
- Allow early return to daily living
- Lower healthcare costs

Factors that determine level of postoperative care after ophthalmic surgery:
- Degree of underlying patient illness (i.e., presence of comorbidities)
- Duration and complexity of the surgical procedure and anaesthesia
- Potential risks of postoperative complications

Time course of postoperative recovery

- Early or immediate recovery: Phase I occurs either in the operative room or the post-anaesthesia care unit (PACU) during which patients emerge from anaesthesia and recover their protective reflexes and motor function.
- Intermediate recovery: Phase II occurs after discharge from the PACU but before discharge home (for ambulatory surgery patients) during which the patient recovers coordination, and physiologic function.
- Late recovery: occurs after discharge from the hospital or the ambulatory surgery facility during which the patient recovers completely from surgery and is ready for routine daily activities.

Throughput after surgery

- Traditional throughput after surgery includes transfer of patients from the operating room to the PACU and then discharge home.
- With improved surgical and anaesthesia techniques many patients are awake, alert, with normal protective reflexes and motor activity, and comfortable in the operating room (i.e., they achieve the PACU discharge criteria in the operating room). Therefore, these patients could bypass the PACU and go directly from the operating room to the phase 2. This approach is referred to as 'fast tracking'.
- Fast tracking allows for rapid throughput and an early discharge, thereby facilitating perioperative efficiency (e.g., shorter stays and reduced costs).

Discharge after surgery

- Discharge from the PACU and discharge home should be clinical-based, not time-based (i.e., there should be no mandatory minimum length of stay).
- Utilization of appropriate scoring systems allows the patients to be safely discharged from the PACU (e.g., modified Aldrete criteria, see Table 23.1) as well as discharged home (e.g., modified post-anaesthesia discharge scoring system, see Table 23.2).
- Patient must have a responsible escort for travel home.

Patient information and education at the time of discharge

- At the time of discharge the post-surgical care should be reviewed with the patient and/or the escort and written postoperative instructions must be provided.
- Importantly, patients must recognize that home-readiness is not synonymous with street fitness.
- Patients must be informed about appropriate signs and symptoms of possible complications, eye protection, activities, medications, required visits, and details for access to emergency care.
- A follow-up appointment should be scheduled.

Table 23.1 Modified scoring system for determining discharge from the post-anesthesia care unit

Activity: able to move voluntarily or on command	
4 extremities	2
2 extremities	1
0 extremities	0
Respiration	
Able to deep breathe and cough freely	2
Dyspnea, shallow or limited breathing	1
Apneic	0
Circulation	
Blood pressure ± 20mmHg of pre-anesthetic level	2
Blood pressure ± 20–50mmHg of pre-anesthetic level	1
Blood pressure ± 50mmHg of pre-anesthetic level	0
Consciousness	
Fully awake	2
Arousable on calling	1
Not responding	0
Oxygen saturation	
Able to maintain SaO_2 >92% on room air	2
Needs supplemental oxygen to maintain SaO_2 >90%	1
SaO_2 <90% even with supplemental oxygen	0

Score ≥9 required for discharge

Table 23.2 Modified post-anaesthesia discharge scoring system for determining home-readiness

Vital signs

	Blood pressure and pulse within 20% of preoperative value	2
	Blood pressure and pulse 20–40% of preoperative value	1
	Blood pressure and pulse >40% of preoperative value	0

Activity level

	Steady gait, no dizziness, or meets preoperative level	2
	Requires assistance	1
	Unable to ambulate	0

Nausea and/or vomiting

	Minimal: successfully treated with oral medication	2
	Moderate: successfully treated with intramuscular medication	1
	Severe: continues after repeated treatment	0

Pain

	Acceptable	2
	Not acceptable	1

Surgical bleeding

	Minimal: does not require dressing change	2
	Moderate: up to two dressing changes required	1
	Severe: more than three dressing changes required	0

Score ≥9 required for discharge.

Postoperative complications

The overall complication rate after ophthalmic surgery remains unknown because the literature is sparse and of limited quality. The mortality after ophthalmic surgery remains significantly low despite of the high-risk population (i.e., American Society of Anesthesiologists Physical Status of III–IV).

Patient-related complications

- Because patients undergoing ophthalmic surgery are usually elderly with numerous comorbidities (see 📖 Changes in the elderly, pp. 188–191), these patient factors contribute significantly to the development of postoperative complications.
- Preoperative hypertension is a risk factor for development of postoperative hypertension and therefore adequate preoperative blood pressure control is critical.
- A study reported that 26% of high-risk patients (e.g., those with diabetes, hypertension) undergoing retinal surgery under LA had at least one silent myocardial ischaemia event within 18h of surgery. However, less than 1% of ophthalmic patients required transfer to medical service.
- Patients who develop significant hypertension and/or tachycardia in the PACU have been reported to have a higher mortality rate.
- Postoperative hypertension and dysrhythmias can also be caused by hypoxaemia, hypercapnia, pain, agitation, bladder distension, and fluid overload as well as increased intra-ocular pressure (IOP) and late manifestations of oculo-cardiac reflex (OCR).
- In diabetic patients, hyperglycaemia can cause dehydration, fluid shifts, electrolyte abnormalities, a predisposition to infection, and impaired wound healing as well as ketoacidosis and hyperosmolar states. Of note, perioperative hyperglycaemia is commonly due to inappropriate discontinuation of preoperative antidiabetic therapy and the perioperative stress response.
- Because many of the patients who are undergoing ophthalmic surgery are elderly who might suffer from prostatic hypertrophy, they may encounter postoperative urinary retention. Although simple in-out bladder catheterization may be adequate, that may prove to be difficult requiring consultation with a urologist.

Regional block and surgery-related complications

- Although most of the complications associated with local/regional anaesthesia techniques can be recognized around the time of block placement, there may be a delay in diagnosis that might occur in the postoperative period.
- Damage to the globe caused by regional block, surgical procedure, and patient movement during surgery is a rare but serious complication, which is usually diagnosed immediately due to intense ocular pain. However, in some cases the signs of globe perforation (e.g., ocular pain) may not occur until the postoperative period.
- Optic nerve injury can be missed during surgery and present in the early postoperative period as marked loss of vision or blindness. The presence of risk factors for optic nerve injury (small orbits, placement of a long

needle deep into apex and the patient looking upwards and inwards at the time of the block) along with marked loss of vision or blindness in early postoperative period requires immediate surgical review.

- Damage to the extra-ocular muscles from orbital blocks can result in diplopia, ptosis, and entropion (i.e., infolding of the lid). Possible mechanisms of this extra-ocular muscle damage include direct needle trauma.

- Ischaemic pressure necrosis caused by a large-volume LA, the direct myotoxic effect of LA on extra-ocular muscle and/or the use of high concentrations of LA.

- Transient diplopia on the first postoperative day is common after eye surgery, however, if it continues beyond the early postoperative period, myotoxicity should be suspected. The most common injury of an eye block is damage to the inferior rectus.

- Ptosis can be caused by dehiscence of the levator aponeurosis due to a large volume of LA, the use of superior bridal stitch or the application of a lid speculum. Ptosis occurs in 50% of cases on the first postoperative day after eye surgery, and resolves in 95% of patients by the fourth postoperative day and in 99% within 5 weeks.

- Late symptoms of an inadvertent LA injection into the subarachnoid or intravascular space (e.g., during the placement of the retrobulbar block) include abnormal temperature regulation, facial paralysis, vomiting, temporary hemiplegia, aphasia, dysphasia, and dysarthria.

- Because complications of OCR (see 🕮 Oculo-cardiac reflex, pp. 44–45) may occur as much as 1–2h after an uncomplicated block, careful monitoring for cardiac arrhythmia should be continued for several hours after retrobulbar block placement.

- Patients receiving a facial nerve block may complain of hoarseness, dysphasia, and laryngospasm, probably due to blockade of the vagus, glossopharyngeal, and spinal accessory nerves that are in the close proximity of the facial nerve. These symptoms may be mistakenly considered as complications related to GA.

- Intra-ocular haemorrhage that is venous in origin has a slow onset and usually presents after surgery as a blood-stained chemosis and raised IOP, and may sometimes require prompt surgical decompression to preserve vision.

- Retinal vascular occlusion (RVO), involving the central retinal artery or both the artery and the vein, is usually diagnosed after surgery. It is caused by injury to the artery during block placement or from the external pressure caused by surgical haemorrhage. Patients with vascular or haematological disease are at a high risk of developing RVO. In this patient population epinephrine-containing LA solutions should be avoided, as they can cause significant reduction in ophthalmic artery pressure.

- Corneal injury may be caused by regional/local block, surgical injury, and general anaesthesia, or could be patient-induced. GA decreases tear production and reduces the normal mechanical eyelid closure. Therefore, it is important to make sure that the eyelids are completely closed to prevent corneal drying due to the absence of blinking and the suppression of lacrimal gland function. The use of non-ionic petroleum-based eye ointment, intraoperatively, as well as preventing the patient from rubbing their eyes postoperatively, may prevent corneal abrasion. The patient who has undergone a local/regional block is at particular risk as the cornea becomes insensitive. Corneal injury is indicated by pain, photophobia and/or a foreign body sensation after surgery and can be confirmed by fluorescein staining of the cornea. The patient should be reassured that a corneal abrasion usually heals and pain relief occurs within 24–48h. Treatment includes topical antibiotics, short-acting cycloplegics, or anti-inflammatory agents as well as covering the eye with a patch. Of note, topical anaesthetics may delay healing and lead to keratopathy, and therefore must be avoided. Rarely, significant corneal reactions, including epithelial defects and stromal ulceration and melting, have been reported with topical ocular NSAIDs.

Sedation/analgesia techniques and general anaesthesia-related complications (see 📖 Postoperative care, p. 149, Complications in PACU, p. 150, Postoperative nausea and vomiting: prevention and therapy, p. 180)

Although the morbidity of sedation/analgesia techniques is low, it can be significant. The complications of sedation/analgesia include:
- Excessive or prolonged somnolence from the residual effects of sedative/hypnotics and opioids, cardiovascular complications such as hypotension and bradycardia, and respiratory complications such as loss of airway patency, respiratory depression, hypoxaemia, and hypercarbia.
- Patients must be carefully triaged to receive an appropriate level of postoperative care by evaluating their status and the potential for complications inherent in the specific procedure.

Others
- Factors that have been associated with postoperative complications include; female gender, no previous exposure to GA, tracheal intubation, abdominal surgery, and surgical time in excess of 20min.
- Adequate preoperative hydration (i.e., avoidance of prolonged fasting and encouraging patients to consume water until 2h prior to surgery) and intraoperative fluid administration may reduce postoperative postural hypotension, dizziness, drowsiness, and nausea.
- Respiratory problems are the most frequently encountered complications in the postoperative period. Patients at risk of these complications include the elderly, the obese and those with obstructive sleep apnoea (OSA). The use of pulse oximetry and capnography may facilitate early detection of these complications.
- Postoperative shivering can occur as a result of intraoperative hypothermia or the effects of anaesthetic drugs. Intense shivering increases oxygen consumption, carbon dioxide production, and cardiac output, which may not be well tolerated by the elderly or those with significant cardiopulmonary disease. Postoperative shivering may be treated with meperidine 10–25mg, IV.
- Hypothermia is associated with an increased incidence of myocardial ischaemia and arrhythmias. Hypothermia in recovery period should be promptly treated with a forced-air warming device.

Complications related to systemic effects of eye medications (see 📖 Ophthalmic medications in children, p. 204, Systemic problems from glaucoma medications, p. 236)

- The eye drops used in the perioperative period may be readily absorbed through hyperaemic conjunctival incision, which can produce a prolonged systemic effect, particularly in the elderly.
- Eye medications that can cause systemic effect in postoperative period include phenylephrine, epinephrine, timolol, echothiophate, acetylcholine, cyclopentolate, scopolamine, and atropine.
- Phenylephrine and epinephrine can cause severe hypertension, arrhythmias, and myocardial ischaemia and therefore should be used with caution in patients with significant hypertension, coronary artery disease and cardiac failure.
- Timolol, a beta-adrenergic receptor blocking drug, can cause bradycardia, hypotension, exacerbation of asthma, and myasthenia gravis.
- Echothiophate drops act systematically to reduce plasma cholinesterase activity and this suppression requires 4–6 weeks to recover after cessation of its use. Patients on echothiophate may have prolonged neuromuscular blockade with suxamethonium.
- Acetylcholine may be used to produce miosis after cataract surgery, and can cause bradycardia, hypotension, bronchospasm, increase bronchial secretion, and salivation.
- Cyclopentolate drops are used to dilate the pupils, and can cause disorientation, dysarthria, and rarely seizures and psychotic reactions.
- Scopolamine eye drops can cause disorientation and hallucinations.

Postoperative pain management

- Effective postoperative pain relief is to be expected and is necessary for improved patient satisfaction.
- The postoperative pain after most ophthalmic surgical procedures is mild to moderate, particularly when the procedure is performed using local/regional anaesthesia technique.
- Some invasive procedures such as vitrectomy with sclera buckling, enucleation or evisceration of an eye, penetrating eye injury, and dacrocystorhinostomy (DCR) may be associated with moderate to severe pain.
- An optimal analgesic technique would consist of a combination of several analgesics that have different mechanisms of action, referred to as a multimodal analgesia technique.
- Oral analgesics should be administered as early as possible postoperatively and preferably preoperatively so that the peak analgesic levels occur before the local anaesthetic wares off.
- The use of a non-opioid technique should reduce opioid requirements and thus opioid-related side effects which include nausea, vomiting, and sedation and may contribute to a delayed recovery and discharge home.
- For procedures with mild to moderate pain, the use of a local anaesthetic technique whenever possible in combination with acetaminophen and NSAIDs or cyclo-oxygenase- (COX-2) specific inhibitors, if there are no contraindications is usually effective.
- For surgical procedures with moderate to severe pain, a combination of acetaminophen, NSAIDs or COX-2-specific inhibitors, and weak opioids (e.g., codeine, hydrocodone, oxycodone) should provide effective pain relief.
- Topical proxymetacaine (proparacaine), a local anaesthetic, eye drops may be used to provide pain relief after cataract extraction, strabismus surgery, and vitreoretinal surgery. However, it is indicated for short-term use only because of the potential for severe corneal damage.
- In patients undergoing DCR surgery, irrigation of the duct with topical LA by the surgeon may contribute to improved pain relief.
- Of note, unusually severe postoperative pain may signal surgical complications such as acute glaucoma, increased IOP, and corneal abrasion.
- Acute glaucoma presents with a severe, diffuse, peri-orbital pain in dry, pale eyes with dilated pupils, without photophobia, tearing, or conjunctivitis. In an acute glaucoma crisis, several drugs from different classes are used simultaneously to accelerate and maximize their pressure lowering effects: topical β-adrenergic agonists (e.g., brimonidine, apraclonidine), β-blockers (e.g., betaxolol, carteolol, levobunolol, timolol), and prostaglandin analogues (e.g., latanoprost).

- Increased IOP is accompanied by reduced vision. Treatment should be aimed at reducing IOP using intravenous mannitol 1gm/kg over 30min or acetazolamide 500mg over 5min. Mannitol might cause hypertension, haemodilution, and acute intravascular volume overload, which could be dangerous in patients with pre-existing cardiovascular diseases. Other measures to decrease IOP may include a head-up position as well as avoidance of direct pressure on the eye, agitation, pain, and increased intravascular volume. In addition, systemic hypertension should be promptly treated.

Postoperative nausea and vomiting

The incidence of postoperative nausea and vomiting (PONV) can be minimized by using prophylactic antiemetics in a patient 'at risk' for developing this complication.

- The risk factors for PONV include female gender, a history of motion sickness, a history of previous PONV, non-smoker status, and the postoperative use of opioids. Other risk factors that are supported by weak evidence include young age, a prolonged duration of surgery, the use of inhalation anaesthesia, and the type of surgical procedure.
- In a similar to multimodal analgesia techniques, multimodal antiemetic therapy (i.e., combinations of 5-HT3-receptor antagonists [e.g., ondansetron], droperidol, dexamethasone, and a scopolamine transdermal patch) is more effective in reducing the incidence and severity of PONV than any single agent.
- This multimodal approach is particularly recommended in patients undergoing strabismus surgery, because PONV remains a common problem after this surgery.
- Antiemetics with different mechanism of action have additive (rather than synergistic) effects. Therefore, the benefit of subsequent antiemetic intervention is less than the initial intervention.
- The number of antiemetics used should be based on the patient's level of risk as determined by risk factor assessment.
- In addition, aggressive perioperative hydration, opioid sparing, and the use of a propofol TIVA technique may reduce the baseline risks of PONV.
- Nausea and vomiting can occur after discharge home (i.e., post-discharge nausea and vomiting [PDNV]). Patients who do not experience PONV prior to discharge home may become symptomatic several hours after discharge when they ambulate, resume oral intake, and consume opioid analgesics. Also, PONV may occur due to the short duration of action of most of the antiemetics and few patients are prescribed antiemetics for home use. Predictors of PONV include female gender, age greater than 50 years, a history PONV, opioid usage, and nausea in PACU. Non-smoking status, intraoperative antiemetics, and types or approaches of surgery were not significant predictors of PONV. Current management options for PONV include the use of oral ondansetron disintegrating tablets and scopolamine transdermal patch.

Postoperative delirium and cognitive decline

- Because a high percentage of patients undergoing ophthalmic surgery are elderly, there is higher likelihood of postoperative confusion or disorientation, delirium, and cognitive decline.
- The presence of pre-existing dementia, cognitive abnormalities, or hearing and visual impairment as well as use of psychogenic drugs predicts postoperative delirium.
- Contributing factors may include sedatives/hypnotics, opioids, and anticholinergics used by ophthalmologists to dilate the pupils as well as the stress of surgery, pain, emesis, sleep deprivation, and a loss of routine.

Delayed discharge after ambulatory surgery

Factors related to delayed discharge from an ambulatory surgery facility include: patient-related factors (i.e., due to comorbidities), anaesthesia and sedation-related factors and surgery-related factors as well as administrative factors (e.g., unavailability of an escort or patient cannot exercise self-care and a responsible adult is not available to stay with the patient).

Unplanned hospitalization after ambulatory surgery

- The incidence of unplanned hospitalization after cataract surgery is reported to be 0.3%. Factors related to unplanned postoperative hospitalization include:

Medical factors

- Cardiac instability (e.g., hypotension, hypertension, and rhythm disturbances)
- Respiratory instability (e.g., airway obstruction, hypoventilation, bronchospasm, and pulmonary aspiration)
- A cerebrovascular episode
- Uncontrolled blood glucose levels requiring acute management
- Uncontrolled nausea or vomiting
- Acute urinary retention
- Significant delirium and cognitive dysfunction

Surgical factors

- Hyphaema
- Uncontrolled elevated IOP
- Threatened or actual expulsive suprachoroidal haemorrhage
- Retrobulbar haemorrhage
- Uncontrolled pain

Post-discharge considerations

- An expectation and therefore a close scrutiny of complications that can occur after discharge from an ambulatory surgery facility is of fundamental importance.
- The most common post-discharge complications are pain and nausea.
- Minor complications after discharge include headache, sore throat and hoarseness, dizziness, drowsiness, myalgia, and syncope, as well as potential side effects of the chronic medications used by the patient, all of which may affect the patient's ability to resume normal activities of daily living.
- Headache remains a common complaint, often persisting for up to 48h after surgery. Headache appears to increase after inhalation anaesthesia. Caffeine withdrawal and fasting are also contributing factors.
- The likelihood of complications is increased significantly when prescriptions were not explained or when the patient is discharged home while in pain or 'feeling poorly'.

Postoperative visit

- The postoperative visit to the surgeon's office/hospital depends upon both patient characteristics and any occurrence of complications.
- Patients that need to be seen within 24h after surgery include high-risk patients, functionally monocular patients, those with glaucoma or who are glaucoma suspect, and patients with intraoperative complications.
- Patients with the presence of risks or signs or symptoms of possible complications should have their first postoperative visit within 48h of surgery to detect and treat early complications, such as infection, wound leak, hypotony, or increased IOP.
- For other patients the visit could be performed 1–4 weeks after surgery.
- The patients should be instructed to contact the ophthalmologist promptly if they experience symptoms such as a significant reduction in vision, increasing pain, progressive redness, or peri-ocular swelling because these symptoms may indicate the onset of endophthalmitis.

Conclusion

There is a significant increase in the number of ophthalmologic surgical procedures annually, across the world. The level of postoperative care necessary after ophthalmic surgery is determined by the degree of underlying patient illness, the duration and complexity of the surgical procedure and anaesthesia, and the potential postoperative risks. Perioperative outcome after an ophthalmic procedure performed on outpatient basis is similar to that performed on an inpatient basis, therefore, the level of postoperative care between inpatients and outpatients should be similar. The goal of postoperative care is to optimize the outcome of surgery through early recognition and management of complications of anaesthesia and surgery. Close scrutiny of complications after discharge is of fundamental importance.

Further reading

Gan TJ. Risk factors for postoperative nausea and vomiting. *Anesth. Analg.* 2006; 102: 1894–8.

Gupta A, Wu CL, Elkassabany N, Krug CE *et al.* Does the routine prophylactic use of antiemetics affect the incidence of post-discharge nausea and vomiting following ambulatory surgery? A systematic review of randomized controlled trials. *Anesthesiology.* 2003; 99: 488–95.

Hamilton RC. A discourse of the complications of retrobulbar and peribulbar blockade. *Can. J. Ophthalmol.* 2000; 35: 363–72.

Joshi G. New concepts in recovery after ambulatory surgery. *J. Amb. Surg.* 2003; 10: 167–70.

Joshi GP. Fast-tracking in outpatients surgery. *Curr. Opin. Anaesthesiol.* 2001; 14: 635–9.

Kumar CM. Orbital regional anesthesia: complications and their prevention. *Indian J. of Ophthalmology.* 2006; 54: 77–84.

Local anaesthesia for intraocular surgery. London: The Royal College of Anaesthetists and the Royal College of Ophthalmologists, 2001.

McGoldrick K and Gayer S. Anesthesia and the eye. In Barash P, Cullen B, Stoelting R, *Clinical anesthesia,* 5th edn. Philadelphia: Lippincott Williams and Wilkins, 2006, pp. 978–95.

Practice guidelines postoperative care. A report by the American Society of Anesthesiologists Task Force on postanesthesia care. *Anesthesiology.* 2002; 96: 742–52.

Stead SW. Complications in ophthalmic anesthesiology. *Seminars in Anesth.* 1996; 15: 171–82.

Conclusion

Further reading

Future developments

Professor Chris Dodds

Introduction

The one constant in clinical care is the change in treatment options which in turn depend on advances in the basic sciences and their integration into novel therapeutic possibilities. This is as true in ophthalmic practice as any other avenue of medicine.

Loss of vision can occur at any age and may be from a wide range of conditions including genetic causes, diseases, age-related degeneration, trauma or malignancy. The loss may be amenable to surgical intervention such as cataract removal or corneal transplantation, or it may be untreatable at the present. The impact that these innovations will have on our practice may be enormous.

All developments start in active academic units where they are tested and where practitioners can learn the necessary diagnostic and practical skills. If they then stand the test of time and rigorous assessment they start to become mainstream practice. This process is becoming faster as simulation allows practice and acquisition of skills often some distance from the host unit.

This roll-out of novel treatments, especially those related to the restoration of sight, is important in the context of the worldwide changes in demography and the relatively greater proportion of elderly.

The importance of restoring vision to enable independent living and improving individual quality of life make this a major health priority across the world and cannot be overemphasized. Restoration of sight enough to be able to navigate around the environment and self-care enables family units to be productive and supportive, whereas caring for a completely dependent relative all too often means one of the earners in the unit have to stop full-time work to provide this care. This is true in the more financially well-off countries as well as those still developing.

As far as ophthalmic practice is concerned there are three major areas of interest that may see great changes in the next 10 years or so. These are:

- Prevention or medical treatment of ophthalmic conditions leading to blindness
- Recovery or replacement of vision
- Enhancement of optical performance

Whist the first may not directly affect surgical ophthalmologists and anaesthetists, the last two certainly will.

Prevention

The prevention of visual loss, in common with most aspects of preventative medicine, is the most cost-effective strategy but also one that depends on a comprehensive public health infrastructure. This is lacking in much of the world and the detailed developments in this area are beyond the scope of this chapter. However, there are aspects that may become part of our everyday practice in the next 10–20 years.

Analysis of the human genome can be expected to lead to genetic therapies either at a pre-conceptual stage, *in utero* or in the postnatal period.

Where the condition is identified to be caused by an intracellular dysfunction, for instance in protein synthesis, this may become a matter for referral to a genetic unit for treatment rather than advice on risks and prognosis. The ability to introduce remedial gene sequences is becoming a proven technology and allows repair or modification of intracellular function. Increasingly these will become identified through routine screening and therapy prescribed.

Acquired visual loss from ophthalmic infections depends on large-scale public health programmes but awareness of the causes, vectors and life-cycle and development and delivery of appropriate antimicrobial/antihelminthic medication may eradicate these preventable causes of loss of vision.

Recovery or preservation

Restoration of sight clearly depends on the underlying cause/s of the visual loss. There are exciting biomechanical, nano-medical and neuro-physiological ventures that will require surgical and anaesthetic expertise in implanting and assessing these devices. The most pragmatic structure to review this is to follow the path of light to the retina and then the neuronal route to the optical cortex.

Anterior segment problems

Corneal damage may follow trauma or infection and whilst many will benefit, as now, from corneal grafting there are those who are unsuitable or who have failed repeated attempts.

Stem cell-culture from traumatized corneas with intact endothelial cells has been successful in restoring full vision after alkali burns, and is likely to become a more routine process where the scarring and damage is not due to primary endothelial dysfunction. Where there is little or no chance of achieving a clear light path to the retina, the implanting of light-emitting arrays behind the cornea or lens, linked wirelessly to an image capture system, can restore a degree of visual function. The potential to use the existing functional retinal bypasses many of the problems inherent in direct retinal stimulation systems, although placement and retention remain potential problems. As with all implants the technical problem of hermetically sealing the electrical devices (and maintaining their function) without causing an inflammatory response or immune response remains to be solved convincingly.

Certainly the *in vivo* studies in rabbits were successful. The question of how to maintain a viable retina in the face of severe globe trauma has not been addressed but for localized anterior damage this is a promising technology using lens extraction and vitrectomy to enable placement as an extension of routine surgical and anaesthetic practice.

Posterior segment problems

Far more common problems occur with the function of the retina, whether this is damage from degenerative diseases such as age related macular degeneration or retinitis pigmentosa (RP) or metabolic ones such as diabetic retinopathy.

One of the key aspects is whether the entire retinal structure is lost or whether it is the surface layers only but with preservation of the ganglion cells.

Various research groups across the world are developing differing methods to restore a degree of sight. Unlike the first device (above) that uses light as the basic signal (as is normally the case) the majority of these use electrical signals with the aim of eliciting phosphenes (visual perceptions not caused by light, often seen as flashes of light).

Before looking at the actual devices some insight into the size of the problem is useful. We process the information arriving at different areas of the retina for differing purposes. Peripheral fields are mostly used to identify moving object within a static field and this function is able to discriminate very small movements within complex visual backgrounds. The macula area provides highly precise processing to help identify objects.

Some 'feature' recognition systems appear to exist across the retina, for faces for example. Being able to navigate through the environment requires an ability to discriminate between static and moving objects within that environment at the same time as recognizing what activity is due to the movement of that individual. This is achieved by a form of parallel processing within the brain.

This complexity of function is affected by retinal disease as well as neurological damage within the central nervous system. To provide an effective bionic replacement it has to match these functions. There are promising computational processing developments that may allow the presentation of electrical signals that will allow the discrimination of movement in real time. The resolution of an electrically induced image depends on the number of pixels the array can provide/generate. The earliest had 16, then 20 and ones with 60 have been reported although the theoretical ideal is over 1000 pixels. They currently need external power sources and an interface to the digital visual capture systems (usually spectacle-mounted video cameras).

The interface may be placed directly unto the damaged retina or placed behind the retina in the episcleral space (sub-Tenon's) The latter position usually allows easier instrumentation and placement but need a greater signal strength.

Retinal transplantation is developing but the technical demands of the surgery and anaesthesia as well as the ability to maintain the placement and adherence of the implant might suggest that the artificial devices are more likely to offer salvage at the moment.

Neuronal level problems

If the retina is completely damaged, stimulation may be directed to the optic nerves or anywhere along the visual pathway, including intracranial placement in the thalamus or over the visual cortex.

Clearly, these developments rely on neurosurgical as well as bio-electrical developments.

Alternative solutions

Another strategy follows the increasing use of nanotechnology. The ability to harvest photosynthetic protein structures and reconstitute them in artificial liposomes has enabled researchers to insert them into mammalian cells which then become reactive to light. This would enable the repair of damaged cells, or more likely the recruitment of undamaged but non-light-sensitive cells, in the retina to restore sight.

The same principle of enabling non-reacting cells to respond to light is used by genetic targeting. One group has injected viral vectors into the vitreous and transfected inner retinal neurons with a microbial-type rhodopsin, Ganglion cells expressing this rhodopsin showed intrinsic light responses.

The impact that this research activity will have on the future of ophthalmic surgical and anaesthetic practice must be to change our practice from attempting to rescue limited sight to providing the best conditions for either implanted artificial retinal prostheses or placement of liposomes, or even thin dye-based membranes. Preservation of the epi-scleral space and avoidance of any possible neuronal/globe damage suggests a return to expertly managed general anaesthesia.

Enhancement

Whilst attempting to restore visual functioning is challenging in its own right, seeking to improve on what has been developed through an evolutionary process is also an attractive goal. If there were to be a true 'bionic' eye why should it be limited to the restricted spectrum of wavelengths we use, the optical acuity of a complex eye or even the field of vision we restrict ourselves to?

The forward-looking placement of our eyes, in keeping with many predators, does enable us to navigate effectively at high speed and avoid hazards at the same time. However, that is simply the result of an evolutionary path and there may be future survival benefits from a full 3D field of view across the radiation spectrum.

The great strides in optical devices have produced very high resolution power from smaller and smaller lens systems at the same time that software and hardware for processing the images are able to utilize these lens systems and filter out artefacts from movement or judder, for instance. Compound eyes can allow simultaneous very long range and ultra-short acuity instantaneously. They could also be specifically tuned to particular wavelengths so that night vision could be as effective as that in daylight.

Neuronal plasticity is able to integrate marked changes in visual signalling into an understandable image even at advanced age. The brain is likely to be able integrate input from high resolution and mixed wavelength devices. The integration between our own biological cellular systems and electronic, chemical or spectral signals could herald the next phase in evolution and one where the equivalent of vision will still be present.

Conclusion

The future for our patients with sight-threatening diseases is improving through the developments in materials science, computing and nanotechnology. Where the current set of knowledge, skills, and attitudes of ophthalmic surgical teams will have to be modified is less clear but change it will have to. Robotic surgery is becoming routine in some surgical fields, prevention of genetically or age-related diseases is being more and more successful. However, the population of the world is getting larger and older day by day. I expect that the demand for high-quality ophthalmic care that we recognize today will be present for at least another 10 years. After that—who knows?

Key reading

Chader GL, Weiland J, Humayun MS. Artificial vision: needs, functioning, and testing of a retinal electronic prosthesis. *Prog. Brain Res.* 2009; 175: 317–32.

Jung GH, Kline DW. Resolution of blur in the older eye: neural compensation in addition to optics? *J. Vis.* 2010; 10(5): 7.

Lagali PS, Balya D, Awatramani GB, *et al.* Light-activated channels targeted to ON bipolar cells restore visual function in retinal degeneration. *Nature Neuroscience.* 2008; 11: 667–75.

Li L and Yi A Y. Development of a 3D artificial compound eye. *Opt. Express.* 2010; 18(17): 18125–37.

Matsuo T, Uchida T, Takarabe K. Safety, efficacy, and quality control of a photoelectric dye-based retinal prosthesis (Okayama University-type retinal prosthesis) as a medical device. *J. Artif. Organs.* 2009; 12(4): 213–25.

Noy A. Bionanoelectronics. *Adv. Mater.* 2011; 23(7): 799.

Pauwels K, Kruger M, Lappe M, Worgotter F, Van Hulle MM. A cortical architecture on parallel hardware for motion processing in real time. *J. Vis.* 2010; 10(10): 18.

Pritchard CD, Arner KM, Langer RS, Ghosh FK. Retinal transplantation using surface modified poly(glycerol-co-sebacic acid) membranes. *Biomaterials.* 2010; 31(31): 7978–84.

Sakaguchi H, Kamei M, Fujikado T, *et al.* Artificial vision by direct optic nerve electrode (AV-DONE) implantation in a blind patient with retinitis pigmentosa. *J. Artif. Organs.* 2009; 12(3): 206–9.

Szurman P, Warga M, Roters S, *et al.* Experimental implantation and long-term testing of an intraocular vision aid in rabbits. *Arch. Ophthalmol.* 2005; 123(7): 964–9.

Zarbin MA, Montemagno C, Leary CJF, Ritch R. Nanomedicine in ophthalmology: the new frontier. *Am. J. Ophthalmol.* 2010; 150(2): 144–62.

Index